I Don't Want to *Be* Old When I Get Old

A Lifestyle Experiment

Thelma J. Lofquist, Ph. D.

First published by AuthorHouse 03/10/05

ISBN: 1-4208-2477-5 (sc)

Library of Congress Control Number: 2005902307

Printed in the United States of America
Bloomington, Indiana

This book is printed on acid-free paper.

Notice of rights

Photos by Lisa Clark and David Hupp

Clip art by *T Maker

For David.

My husband, lover, friend and editor. Without you our book would never have been finished.

Although I still believe I can use "plethora" if I want to.

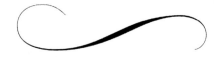

About the cover:

I have fun riding around on a grocery cart while shopping with my husband. We had gone to a store to buy the kind of apple cider that comes in a champagne bottle. The cranky checkout clerk, never looking at me, said: "If there's alcohol in that you have to show me some ID." I said: "Uh, it's apple cider." She picked up the bottle, looked at it, slammed it down and said: "You're OK then." David said, "Go back and show her your ID." But I kept walking because what she had said made no sense. I was 65 years old! I tried to compare her demeanor with a waiter who kids around, saying: "You have to show me some ID young lady." But this clerk wasn't kidding.

Finally, I concluded that she must have seen us playing around on the grocery cart and had not looked at me closely when I was at the checkout stand.

The incident certainly demonstrates that the way our bodies move through space tells more about our age than does the actual number of years lived.

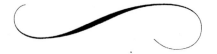

Contents

"We only get one life — this I know
I want to get my licks in now before I go."
—Dire Straits

vi

*I*ntroduction

I DON'T WANT TO BECOME FRAIL AND DEPENDENT, ever. I don't want to ride a bus to Canada to get prescriptions filled. I don't want to need prescriptions. I cannot tolerate the thought of depending upon a stranger to cut my toenails.

I shudder when someone tells me that "so and so" just died. "Don't you remember? You sent her to my care home 13 years ago."

Thirteen years living in a care home, her immediate environment one or two rooms. My immediate environment is the mountains to the east and the coast to the west. I can be in one place or the other in little over an hour *and* be able to go whenever I choose.

It's not the added years I fear; it's the frail dependency, losing mental acuity, sitting in a wheelchair at age 104 celebrating a birthday in a care facility, while everyone is saying, "isn't she beautiful?" Beautiful is the ability to rise from that wheelchair and walk away from the care center.

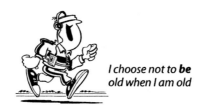

*I choose not to **be** old when I am old*

1

Choice

I choose not to *be* old when I am old.

Choice nudged me into becoming my own research project. If the studies are correct in assuming that lifestyle is a major part of how we age, then the design of my own later years should depend on choosing a healthy, active lifestyle. We are told that frail, dependent aging as well as health problems are preventable. But prevention requires concentrated, realistic planning and, more importantly, it takes determination coupled with patience. It is possible to make that choice.

As a graduate student I taught classes on physical activity and aging. The light began to dawn during those classes. Research suggested it was possible to sidestep the ravages of frail, dependent aging by the way we live.

The final push came as I worked in the field, assessing care facilities. I knew I would never want to live in one.

Ironically, choice was a major feature in most of my training. However, it was a different concept of choice, because the message was: When people are old and frail they should be allowed to have as much choice over their decisions and lifestyle as possible. "Allowed" is the key word here.

A study published at least 25 years ago is still quoted today as a prime example of the benefit of "choice" for seniors. A nursing home was the site. The

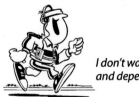

*I don't want to become frail and dependent, **ever.***

2

resident population of two floors were fairly equal in distribution of disabilities. Each resident on one floor was given a plant from a large box and told the nurse would care for it. They were also told that a certain night was movie night and someone would come and escort them.

The residents on the second floor were shown a box of different plants and told they could pick one out if they wished, but they would need to care for it themselves. They were told there would be a movie night; they could decide among themselves which night; they would have a choice of movies; and they could go if they wished. I believe there was an attempt to put tape on the wheels of wheelchairs to see who traveled about the nursing home the most, but the difficulty in measuring the dirt collected on the wheels became a problem.

The study intended to demonstrate that by offering nursing home residents more choices they would become more sociable. As expected, more of the residents who had some control participated in activities, visited with other residents and went actively about the nursing home, compared to the residents who were not given choices. And this research has long been used as an example of demonstrating the benefits of giving choices to older people.

This study has been so overused with such ferocity that I have seen families and social workers offering choices to extremely frail victims of advanced dementia. The study claims that older people are better off if they can continue to make their own life choices, and I agree. But the concept of "old" ought not be the criterion; rather, the criterion should be their state of mind or the care and attention they require. Many times I have been called upon to try and convince someone to move from their residence when they are a danger to themselves and others. I can't convince that dependent person because they won't let me in and the family is wringing their hands and agreeing with the doctor that they should have the right to stay where they are until they "choose" to move.

I have seen older people who are mentally competent, but physically their bodies are a mess, expecting services from family, friends or social agencies that cannot be met. Yet the rallying cries are: "We must give them the choice." "We may die or have a nervous breakdown, but they have the right." "We promised to never put them into a nursing home."

Or, even worse, I have seen frail people who can barely walk or see only with difficulty climb into an automobile, drive off on the wrong side of the road, around a corner and their family says, "We just cannot take that car away. It's their independence." That poor choice has had terrible consequences for those innocent victims who have been run down by elders claiming their independent right to drive.

When closely examining the word "choice" in aging, we must consider the word "allow." It makes perfect sense to "allow" nursing home residents to choose a plant or movies. It is the *nice* thing to do for nursing home quality of life. But "allowing" driving while dangerous, or "allowing" living in urine, developing sores, with the possibility of burning a house down

4

is a different matter. My mother, bless her heart, got a ticket for driving too slowly when she was seventy. She said, "That's it." She gave up her car and quit driving.

I do not want to drive if I am experiencing difficulty with my reflexes and my sight. I do not want to live independently if I can't clean myself properly or remember to turn the stove off.

But, more important, I want to maintain responsive reflexes as long as possible. I want to be able to use the bathroom, finish the job and not smell bad. I want to cut my own toenails until I leave this earth. I want to be able to *recognize* my toenails.

I want to be able to go to the beach or the mountains or to Europe when I choose. I don't want to live for 13 years in a care home. I want to read books and magazines and understand what they are saying. I want friends and family to visit me because they like conversing with me or enjoy being in my company, not because it's a duty and they feel sorry for me.

Choices must be made early on, long before we are in a place where we are "allowed" choices. And I want to demonstrate the long-term value of making lifestyle choices that allow for a viable older age.

The Research Project

When I was much younger I believed, as many young people do now, that older people never seemed to have

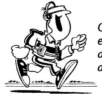

Choices must be made early on, long before we are in a place where we are "allowed" choices.

5

much fun and being very old was the end of life. You could not go many places or appear to want to.

Old age was not on my mind until I entered a university at age 37.

At that time funds were available for the new discipline of Gerontology and the subject seemed a wise choice. Along the way I taught classes on physical activity and aging and there was plenty of evidence, even then, to indicate that caring for both mind and body was beneficial for the aging process.

The term "Successful Aging" evolved from research funded by the MacArthur Foundation, where the lifestyles of hundreds of older adults were examined in great detail. Those deemed "successful" elders were physically active, involved in life, and content. Aging was divided into the categories of "old" and "old/old." Even the "old/old" could be classified as successful if they were living independently, were mentally active, and reasonably satisfied with life. It seemed that one could make a choice to be successful in old age. That is, if the fickle finger of fate didn't hand you a bad apple, such as a genetic disorder or a catastrophic accident.

The more recent evidence seems to convey that even some poor genetic or environmental bad apples can be sidestepped. If there is a family history of strokes and heart attacks, the right lifestyle can be a preventative. Even family histories of some cancers can be avoided with the proper diet and exercise.

And in the past few years the exciting research concerns the plasticity of our brains. We can generate new brain cells at any age, something that was considered impossible for so long. We can activate new neural pathways. And some people can avoid the debilitating problems of Alzheimer's even when their brains seem damaged.

I want a healthy brain. And I also want what most of us hope for: We hope to live a long time with strong bodies and active, alert minds. I believe that we all entertain some hope of living until 100, hauling water and chopping wood, and dying quietly in our sleep.

And news stories abound describing octogenarians running marathons and lifting weights. I don't particularly want to lug water buckets or chop wood or run a marathon. I do want to lift weights, play basketball, read a good book, go to restaurants, travel, and make love. As I informed my husband early in our relationship, what I wanted from him was laughing, sex, and hanging out — not necessarily in that order, just jumbled all together in basket and pulled out randomly. And I fear that if I *am* old, when I am old, I won't be able to pull those treasures from the basket.

The Design

A major part of my research is to do those things that I have learned make for healthy, vital, later years. I've learned extensively from years of going to school, from working with the elderly, from reading everything available about healthy aging, and from living.

I exercise six days a week, with both weight work and aerobics. I eat a reasonably healthy diet. I keep my mind active with reading, word games, taking classes, socializing with family and friends, writing, traveling, and making love.

I get a complete physical every year, measuring cholesterol, blood sugar levels and bone density, and examining hearing and eyesight.

Principles

My fitness principles are discussed chapter by chapter:

- Something must inspire us to get started.
- A good sense of our bodies is vital because everything we do regularly affects our bodies.
- Pleasure and habit must be integrated into a fitness regimen.
- Aerobics are needed for healthy hearts and circulation.
- Muscle building is necessary for strength and bone density.
- Flexibility keeps joints fluid and allows us move about with ease.
- Keeping our brains active prevents us from *being* old, when we are old.
- Healthy eating benefits the brain as well as the body.

When I feel lazy about going to the gym I only need to visit a care center or even a retirement facility to get my attitude corrected. The people who live there are my epiphany.

My regimen is such a habit that my brain tells my body it doesn't feel right if it doesn't get some exercise and vegetables every day. I make it a point to regularly eat certain foods and am active enough to be able to eat what I please. Avoiding rich food has become such a habit that I don't feel tempted. I play mind games and enjoy myself while exercising and love shooting basketball hoops with my husband and grandchildren.

I just received a pleasure hit. A young man at my gym was using a triceps-building machine at 95 lbs. and sighed as he got off, saying. "This workout stuff gets hard at times." I said, "Yeah, but isn't it fun being stronger than most people?" Then I upped the weight to 120 lbs. His look was my joy.

I know that what is going on in my head keeps me going.

"I treat my body like a temple
You treat yours like a tent."
— J. J. Cale

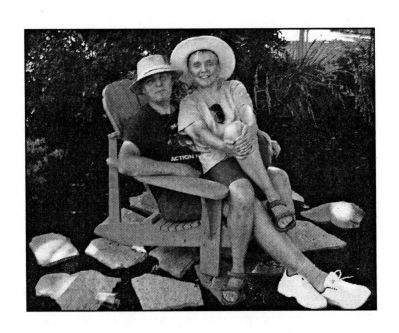

1 *Lifestyle*

I USED TO BELIEVE THAT HALF of nursing home residents would not have needed to be there had they known what to do about healthy living and done it. I thought that genetics was 50% responsible for their frailties.

Now studies indicate that genetics accounts for a much smaller percentage of how we become when we are old. The MacArthur Foundation research came up with 37% and a more recent study claims that genetics accounts for only 17% of older age disabilities.

When we first come into the world our genes do account for most of the way we are. Environment in the womb, how our mother lived and ate had an impact but our genes were the big decider. As we grow and age the environment and our lifestyle begins to entwine with our genes and act on our bodies and our brains. Most of those born with terrible genetic problems die off before they become old. How and where we live becomes more of a deciding factor in our health and mobility and disposition the older we become.

*"We all want a long life,
we just don't want to get old"*
— Chinese Proverb

As an example:

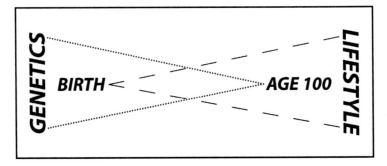

The value on our physical makeup of exercise and eating well has been known for a long time. Magazines abound with information on certain foods as anti oxidants to counter unhealthy aging. The research is continuing all the time with more and more information available on the value of healthy eating.

The same goes for regular exercise. Studies of healthy older adults all indicate how valuable regular physical activity is in sustaining strength and mobility. And more and more we see those successfully aged, active, healthy older people who are involved with life.

But when we visit a medical clinic or hospital or even a shopping mall, we can see how many older people experience difficulties. We watch television programs that feature the impact of prescription costs on older people and see all those elderly piling on a bus to get into Canada to buy their medicines.

A majority of older adults suffer physical health problems. Their later years not only aren't blessed with "golden," they are the most difficult years of their lives.

Even more significant are the more recent studies on our brains. Gone are the old ideas of our being born with a given quantity of brain cells and that the cells that die with age are not replaced. We seem to be able to generate new cells. We not only can generate new cells, we can build new pathways. If a brain is damaged due to a stroke and part of a body is paralyzed, a different area of the brain can be stimulated to develop pathways so motion in paralyzed limbs can be regenerated.

For the rest of us who are concerned about our later years, substantial research that indicates stimulating our brains with mental activity helps postpone mental decline. The most telling evidence is one example of an elderly nun in David Snowdon's book *Aging With Grace*. Dr. Snowdon's ongoing, long term research with elderly nuns who have donated their brains for the study of Alzheimer's disease tells of Sister Bernadette, who did extremely well in the yearly cognitive mental tests right up to her death of a heart attack at age 84. At no time did she ever show any behavioral signs of mental decline or dementia. Yet the autopsy of her brain revealed severe plaques and tangles, all an indication of a brain giving out many years earlier. The differences between the autopsied brain and the mental tests surprised the researchers. The only explanation was of a woman who resisted the symptoms of Alzheimers by keeping her brain active. This surprising result turned up several times with some of the sisters who demonstrated mental sharpness in spite of damaged brains.

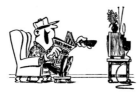

A majority of older adults suffer physical health problems. Their later years are not only not blessed with "golden," they are the most difficult years of their lives.

New research indicates that regular physical activity not only stimulates our brains, it aids in developing new brain cells. Just asking older adults to learn to balance on one leg sets the brain on fire.

Want to begin stimulating your own brain? Move your computer mouse to your opposite hand. Go for a walk and dribble a basketball with one hand. Then on the return, dribble the basketball with the other hand.

Learn to read music. Do puzzles. Exercise regularly. Learn to dance.

Life is short. Our body is our carrying case, the person we are is in that case, and there is only one way out. We don't want to be trapped in a carrying case that hurts. We want a body that functions well and feels good, and we want it to be that way for a long time. Barring accidents and the "fickle finger of fate" our bodies will do just that if we make the right life choices.

The older we are, the greater the impact of our lifestyle is on both our physical and mental health. The old adage of "what we don't use, we lose" is still holding up.

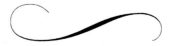

When we first come into the world our genes account for most of the way we are. Environment in the womb — how our mother lived and ate — had an impact but our genes were the big decider. As we grow and age the environment and our lifestyle begins to act on our bodies and our brains. Most of those born with terrible genetic problems die before they become old. How and where we live becomes more of a deciding factor in our health and mobility and disposition the older we become.

2 *Life Is An Exercise*

YOUR MOTHER WAS RIGHT:
Your face will freeze that way.

Joints freeze from lack of motion in the bodies of people living sedentary lives. Bodies freeze as they move stiffly and rigidly through space. Some people's bodies freeze into the shape of a couch. Facial expressions become locked. Chronic pain, frowns, and perpetual disapproval etch into expressions. Walking becomes methodical plodding. Shoulders become hunched over when you are tired, or clenched when you are tense. This freezing, this forming of bodies, does not necessarily wait until age 85; it can happen by age 40, and even earlier.

So many of us pay little or no attention to our bodies or how we physically feel until we are brought up short by pain or illness. The way we move constantly shapes us: How we stand; how we sit; the expressions on our faces; and, most important, how we feel. The first step in any exercise program requires sharpening our body sense, something easier said than done.

A good sense of body makes it easier to find pleasure in the doing. Eventually looking like a picture perfect model is not part of any guarantee. Moving through life, enjoying how your body feels, are results you can count on.

The Mind & Body Connection

Mind and body are intimately connected.

We know that what goes on in people's heads can affect their physical health. We can lower heart rate and blood pressure with biofeedback. We can visualize peaceful places in our minds to ease pain, heal more quickly from surgery and, in some cases, make ourselves well. Evidence indicates that the mind is also a factor in making us sick. Depression reduces immune system capability. Constant anger affects the health of our hearts.

The reverse also seems to be true. It is possible to change emotions by changing how our bodies move. Women who must walk alone in either an unfamiliar or isolated place are advised to move deliberately and look confident. Stalkers and other predators look for hesitant, shy women as victims. Evidence suggests that forcing the body to walk in a sure, strong manner will help a hesitant woman feel strong and firm inside.

A small research project indicated that when subjects would force a smile while depressed, their spirits would lift. Try it: It's worth a test. I look into a mirror and smile, then I say, "Poor me, I suffer so." This game usually causes me to laugh at myself.

Body Sense

We can sharpen our perception of our own mind/body connection by developing a conscious feeling for our body and how it works.

One tactic in learning to develop body sense is to become aware of how our bodies can form themselves and how others have shaped themselves over time. The mall is a good place to begin observing other people. Go sit for awhile and watch faces. You will see younger faces with the beginnings of set expressions and older ones with those expressions etched in. Expressions that most fascinate me are the perpetually disapproving faces. After watching faces, begin to notice bodies. Notice how stiff some people's bodies move, almost as if their joints were frozen. But be somewhat discreet and try not to stare as you watch. This is supposed to be an unobtrusive learning experience.

Even physically active people may not develop well without a sense of their own bodies. I often watch people as they work out in fitness centers. One particular young woman has fascinated me with that look of perpetual disapproval etched into her face. As she watches herself in mirror, the look disappears — she doesn't know it's there. What if that young woman in the gym would exercise and eat right all her life and reached age 85 in perfect physical health yet, because her demeanor seemed too unfriendly, no one would want to go near her or spend time with her? It could happen. It does happen.

I recall a favorite professor coming to class showing a look of astonishment because he had caught a glimpse of himself in a mirror as he approached in the hall. He had wondered who that grouchy-faced person was, until he realized it was himself. He said, "I don't think I feel that way. I looked scary." Only

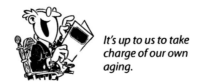

It's up to us to take charge of our own aging.

he knew what thoughts were going through his head that caused that constant look of anger to etch onto his face. But he is a prime example of how our bodies do become etched without our knowledge.

Concentrating on how you move, stand, sit, and feel may appear to be self-engrossed, and it is, because it is necessary to learn about your body; but it's not egotistical. Compare how self-absorbed you become when you are sick or hurt.

My husband's father was an accountant all his life, working hunched over paperwork. When he retired, he continued to hunch over his typewriter while writing. As he aged, his body became frozen in that position, his back deeply curved forward, his hands stiffened and frozen close to his chest. His esophagus had dropped down into his stomach and his stomach acid often burned up into his esophagus. He was scrunched into constant pain for many years. Eating became difficult. His hunched-over posture adversely affected his nerves and he lost feeling throughout his body, particularly his extremities.

Another example: I had observed a new client as I approached to meet her. I did not need to be a psychologist to recognize someone walking along in a deep depression. And she had a right to be depressed, because her husband had recently died. She had not been married long, the marriage had been the best part of her life, and she grieved. But, ten years later,

The first step toward healthier living is sharpening our body sense: How we walk, how we sit, how we move through life. Everything we do with regularity, whether positive or negative, impacts on our bodies.

18

she still walked as a person in a deep depression. She had never followed through with plans she had talked about — traveling and becoming involved with children. Her body, along with her life, was frozen into that deep, deep depression.

It is possible to change how you feel by changing how your body moves. Try smiling when you feel low; standing a little straighter; or walking a tad more briskly.

You want your body to transport you, with ease and good feeling, wherever you go. The ease of movement and lack of pain are the beautiful side effects of a physically active lifestyle.

Gravity Works On You

Want to watch and feel the force of gravity on your body?

First thing in the morning, measure your height. Just before you go to bed, measure your height again in the same way. You will find you are shorter in the evening. Gravity is a powerful force as we move through life.

Notice the necks of older adults. Check yourself and you will find two rather flat muscles in the front of your neck. Behind those muscles are two cords. As you shorten over time, so does your neck, the flat muscles lose tone and those cords are forced to fall forward.

Before you go to bed, stand up straight, feet apart equal to the width of your hips, weight slightly forward on the balls of your feet. Mentally attach an eye bolt to the top of your head, attach the eye bolt to a piece of fairly strong elastic. The other end of the elastic you mentally attach to the ceiling. The elastic should feel not too loose, nor too taut. Mentally feel the pull

19

upward. Then gently pull your shoulders down while continuing to feel the upward pull. If you have never done this before you can develop sore muscles down your neck, so be gentle with yourself. If you do it right, however, you are lengthening your neck.

Another isometric exercise for the neck is to slightly tip your head back as you are driving or riding uphill. Keep your eyes on the road. Too far back hurts the back of your neck. There will be a slight pressure on those flat muscles.

Standing up straight when you are feeling dumpy can become a habit. Walking briskly when you would rather lag can become another habit. It takes effort to move like that when you don't feel energetic inside, but it's worth the effort.

Just by learning to pay attention to how you move through space and altering how you walk and stand and sit will not only make major changes in how you look when you are older, it will be a powerful force in how you feel about yourself.

Bone cells change as constantly as skin and we can take advantage of this fact. We can act to preserve our bone density and keep our bodies flexible.

A dear friend suffered mightily as her bones lost their ability to support her weight — they had lost some of their calcium. I still recall the sadness on her doctor's face as he tried to explain to her that her pain was caused by her crumbling ribs, and that those failing ribs would eventually heal in that deformed position.

Calcium loss in sedentary nursing home patients can be measured in their urine — calcium in, calcium out. In such patients more calcium is eliminated than is taken in. Add more calcium to the diet, more calcium comes out. We literally can lose our bones through our urine as our bones lose density.

What keeps bones dense? One factor is getting enough calcium. But the most important action we can take to protect our bones is to hold onto the calcium we already possess and take in naturally in our diet. Bones keep their density with movement, exercise and muscle buildup. Muscles attached to bones force bones to hang on to the calcium. Moving your body and working on muscles avoids crumbling bones and pain.

And loss of flexibility makes the problem worse. Rigid ligaments accompany bone loss, as well as reducing flexibility. As flexibility in ligaments and other connective tissue decreases, joints stiffen. When joints have stiffened, they not only ache, they are prone to injury. Stiff joints contain little natural synovial fluid. Without that fluid, a sudden move that a younger person could do easily would hurt an older person with a stiff joint. Those stiff joints create a rigidity that can cause the adjoining bones to break more easily upon impact or stress than would the bones in a more flexible body.

The secret to sustaining both flexibility and bone density? Keep on moving! Because of rigidity, many people become less able to turn or move quickly. Whenever my 97 year-old grandfather stepped sideways, he would feel dizzy — it's an example of the

You could amuse your friends at parties by whirling for 30 minutes. Of course, you could discover more practical ways to develop balance and agility.

lightheadedness many older adults experience when they turn or stand quickly. Sometimes that dizziness causes a fall and the resulting broken hip that never heals.

When children play, they run, they turn, they whirl. A five year old loves to spin. As we age we tend to turn less and less and gradually we lose the ability to turn without getting dizzy.

Yet 80- and 90-year-old whirling dervishes in India spin with ease. So do many dancers and ice skaters, including older people who practice these activities regularly. They spin and when they stop, they not only do not fall over, they're not dizzy.

One possible way to begin a lifestyle change might be to travel to India, locate a whirling guru and learn to spin. Then, when you are 90 years old and someone taps you on the shoulder, you will spin around with ease. As an added benefit, you could amuse your friends at parties by whirling for 30 minutes. Of course, you could find more practical ways to develop balance and agility, such as taking a dance class.

We all possess a certain set of genes and a body type. Some people enjoy a natural balance and agility. Most of us must concentrate and work hard on developing our balance and agility in order to move our bodies with relative ease. But whatever body type we have, maintaining agility produces enormous benefits later in life.

Before you begin working on any lifestyle changes, pay special attention to what your body is trying to tell you. Ask yourself: Is it possible to walk a bit more briskly, or improve your posture? Would your body rest easier if you stretched a little before bed? Be courageous. Experiment a little. Listen to what help is offered. Know yourself. Confidently think about what you like and dislike. Try to identify and locate what exercises fit you and your capabilities. Remember that you are unique.

Negative genetic influences can be altered by our lifestyles, just as positive genetic traits can be compromised if our lifestyle is harmful. You are unique in that carrying case — your body — and you don't want it to hurt. You want it to last a long, long time.

It is important to remember our individuality as we become more aware of our bodies and what we can do with them. None of us hears a piece of music exactly the same as another. It's not that some people march to different drummers; rather, we each march to our own drum. So we may as well accept and enjoy our differences.

Expanding on the thought of our differences, it's entirely possible that no one person perceives any given event exactly like anyone else. Don't fall for so-called cookie-cutter or one-size-fits-all programs — what pleases someone else may not please you.

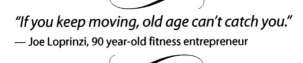

"If you keep moving, old age can't catch you."
— Joe Loprinzi, 90 year-old fitness entrepreneur

We are unique in our carrying cases — our bodies — and we don't want to hurt. We want to last a long, long time. But, waiting in a clinic or watching people at a mall, it doesn't take long to realize how few of us have any real sense of our bodies. It usually takes an illness or accident before we pay attention. Then it may be too late. Developing a body consciousness — how we move through space, how we sit, the expressions on our faces — is a major step in lifestyle change.

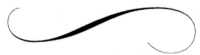

3 *Have An Epiphany*

EPIPHANIES ARE WONDERFUL THINGS. They cause an "aha!" light go on in your head and propel you toward life changes. They can give you a jump start on new or old ideas. Yet many epiphanies just don't last long enough.

Witness the New Year's resolutions that carry over no further than a month or two. You start enthusiastically, ride the momentum, then stagger and stop. Even more serious are the negative physical traumas like heart attacks, mild strokes, and diagnoses of diabetes. Those experiences are potential epiphanies and should produce enough of a jump start into healthier eating and regular exercise. For some, they are powerful motivators; for others, they're like New Year's resolutions. The momentum builds, then the epiphany falters and quits.

If 95% of patients with imminent health problems, who have been advised by their doctors to begin a regular exercise program, do not follow that advice then the thought of improved health, or even the avoidance of early death is not enough of an epiphany to change a sedentary lifestyle. Either no light went on in their heads or, if it did, they were denying they had a problem.

My husband, David, tells a story about himself as a young man. As he sat smoking after dinner during a church potluck he began conversing with the woman sitting next to him. Bothered by his smoke, she removed some pictures of her deceased husband's autopsied "smoker's lungs" from her purse to show to David and make a point about the dangers of smoking. David looked at the pictures with interest while lighting up a new cigarette from the one he hadn't yet finished. A beautiful example of denial. The photos were sad and disgusting but apparently he felt they had nothing to do with his life.

A most shocking example of wasted epiphanies comes from the University of Pittsburgh's studies of a group of smokers who had received heart transplants. Thirty eight percent of the smokers relapsed, half of those within two months of the transplant. One smoker started up the next day. The gift of a new heart and a chance at continuing life wasn't enough of an epiphany to propel a those smokers into changing.

Personal Epiphanies

Some epiphanies can exert such a powerful impact on our minds that they stay with us for years. When I was a child I would watch my elderly aunts, fascinated by their bickering and criticism. I heard them fight many times about who should do what part of the housework. I would say to myself, "When I grow up, I don't want to be like that."

I'm fortunate in having been provided a steady and continuous supply of experiences that have reinforced my lifestyle goals because I have visited elder care homes several times a month for many years. "When I grow up, I don't want to be like so many of the elders whose minds are good, but whose bodies are frail and dependent."

I think about a friend who spent her last years in a nursing home. Her mind was alive and active, and she would have loved to move to a smaller care home where she could have had a private room. But she was so heavy she needed to be lifted with a specialized Hoyer lift. Thus her needs required nursing home care.

As older adults become less physically able and their surroundings shrink, their immediate environment shrinks to the area around their bed. My late mother-in-law went from living the love of artistically arranging a vast organic garden to settling for arranging a vase of flowers from her garden in her bedroom as she became frail. "I don't want my life to shrink to a vase of flowers."

When I was an administrator in a retirement facility I used to wonder about residents who sat and listened to the water in the pipes. It became their focus and they complained about it. When you can't leave the room, everything about it becomes important. Environments not only shrink, so does that list of important things. "I don't want my life reduced to complaining about noisy pipes."

Even the healthiest of us will see our reachable environments shrink as we age. Someday I may not be able to take myself to the coast or the mountains, but I hope I still will be able to go for a walk.

Finding your epiphany
Epiphanies come to each of us in so many different ways. Those revelations can come in small steps or big jumps.

My husband's exercise epiphany was much different than mine. David says:

"My epiphany came in small steps. I started to exercise and was feeling better, but the "aha" came when Latin jazz master Tito Puente died. He had played in our town a couple of years ago and I had wanted to go and take my wife. But I didn't even mention to her that I wanted to do this because I didn't have the stamina to dance. When he died I lost my chance to hear and dance to him again. The light went on — I was determined to never again lose an opportunity like that. I really wished I had had the stamina to dance one more time to this marvelous band.

"Later that year I got another boost. A news story described a man who had been working with an athletic trainer for 3 years to improve his posture, strength and confidence. At the beginning, his trainer said, 'he had an old person's shuffle — bent over, barely lifting his legs.' After the 3 years this man competed in a Nike World Masters Games track and field meet and set a world record for the shot put in his age class. You see, he was 103 by that time. He inspired me, because I figured if a 100 year-old guy can begin a workout routine, so can I!"

For my friend Tim, the exercise epiphany came in his 30s when he realized that all the men in his family had died in their early 50's or late 40's. He wanted to see his children and grandchildren grow up. He says, "I know I have to die, I just don't want to die early like a lump on the couch."

When I told the mid-aged lawyer who works out at my gym about the 95% of people who are told to exercise to save their lives, but don't do it, he said: "I exercise because I don't want to look like that 95%. If I didn't work out my stomach would be huge."

Another friend with fibromyalgia starting exercising gently and steadily when she found the exercise reduced her pain. Her illness became her epiphany.

Tony, a long-time friend I had met at a gym many years ago, said he had discovered his epiphany when he read a thesis relating health and spirituality.

I interviewed a 60 year-old, strong-looking woman at my fitness center. She said she works out much like I do. She revels in her strength. While using a weight machine she concentrates on the muscles she is working and is fully aware of how strong they are. Fear of osteoporosis got her started. Pleasure in her accomplishments keeps her going.

On a more serious note, Jack, who also works out regularly at the gym, had always been an athlete who loved exercise and body building. He was training for a triathlon on his bicycle when he crashed and flew over the handlebars. His injuries literally left him a quadriplegic. He recovered enough to be able to walk with crutches and use a "City Bug" electric cart to move around town. He exercises now for therapy to help himself get through the day. He struggles to reach and use each machine, but he does it. Some days are more difficult than others and his workout might make him feel better for an hour. Other days the effect will last for 6 hours.

Jack is truly my exercise hero: The effort he must exert to stay with his exercise regimen impresses me deeply.

You can see the differences in why people exercise. A minister tells me he works out because he believes his body is a temple for the holy spirit. He says, "I want to have the best temple possible."

Nurturing Your Epiphany

I am going to assume that readers of this book have had a beginning breakthrough. Something has propelled you into knowing that a regular exercise program is necessary in your life and you are exploring ways to make that happen. Becoming fully aware of your epiphany experience is the first step in using your mind to keep you exercising.

However, in order to keep that light burning in your head, it is necessary to nurture the epiphany. You might talk about it, you can talk to it, you could turn it over and over in your head. It simply must not be allowed to go away.

Put pictures or printed quotations (your own or others') up in your bathroom about your epiphany. Watch for people who are experiencing whatever it is you hope to avoid. Talk to yourself about it. Look in a mirror and talk about it. If it's a negative physical epiphany that has propelled you, let it scare you.

Most of us hope to live a long life, but the goal of a healthy older age will not motivate us to start and stay with a fitness regimen. Old age is like death: It's going to happen someday, just not now.

Emotions give our experiences energy. Allow yourself to feel your emotions fully around your epiphany. If it is positive, feel the great joy in it. if it is negative, let it scare you into action.

After many, many months of regular exercise, when you are experiencing the benefits of what you are doing for your body, you can let up a little on the fear aspect.

My epiphany, which has worked well for me, still needs steady upgrading. Even though I truly enjoy how my body moves through space, I sit and observe stiff, tight bodies and know how easy it would be to have a similar body if I didn't keep moving.

Exercise Is A State Of Mind

The key missing move, between "knowing we should get fit" and "doing it," is what is exactly what can be found in our heads.

Even though most of us hope to live a long life, the goal of a healthy older age is not motivation enough to start and stay with a fitness regimen. Old age is like death: It's going to happen someday, just not now.

If we want to reap its benefits, exercise must be frequent and become a long-term habit. Benefits will happen; we just must dance through the maze of difficulties we encounter to get there. It's the "doing it" that's the problem.

After the starting jolt we need new perspectives on how we regard our bodies. Then we need new goals.

 Most of us require a jump start to change and improve our lifestyles. Whatever that something is, we must nurture it to get our minds on track and to keep the motivation from slipping away.

How long does it take to get fit? My postmaster joined a gym and began going three times a week, doing aerobics on a stationary bike and weight work on the machines. He went faithfully for three months. He said he had always had a problem with cutting the grass on a large piece of property he owned that required mowing several times a year. The job was so hard he would stop and rest at least three times before he was finished. After his gym stint of three months he was surprised when he went to do the mowing. That man not only did not need to rest, he was not even tired when he finished.

Three months for some people, three years for others: It depends on how faithfully fitness begins to figure in our lives.

The famous and popular brain doctor, neurologist Richard Restak, writing about the connection between fitness and brain health, says: "You do the fitness often enough and something marvelous happens. You and the fitness become one. Finally, the fitness does you."

If getting started on making fitness a part of your life is difficult you begin by changing what is going on in your head, and finding something that will help you stay focused on change. Fitness truly is a state of mind.

It helps to jump start lifestyle changes if an "aha" light goes on in our heads. But the problem with most epiphanies is that they don't last long enough. Witness the New Year's resolutions that fall by the wayside. When we have an epiphany we have to nurture it. Keep it by our sides. Post it on the bathroom mirror. If necessary, let it scare us. Then when the healthy lifestyle habit kicks in we can ease up a little.

4 First Goal Is Pleasure

AFTER A SMACK ON THE PSYCHE, we tend to make goals and promises to ourselves. However, the goal of "exercising so we will be healthy" when we are old will fizzle because old age is too far away. Most of us foresee old age as most of us envision death. It's going to happen sometime, just not now.

The goal of a buff body usually doesn't work either. Body development doesn't happen fast enough and most of us are too far from perfection. Taking precious time out of every day to exercise for some "pie in the sky results" won't last for the long term. The epiphany momentum staggers and stops because the object of our efforts is so far away.

Our goals must be realistic. We are creatures of the moment. That reality can help us exercise regularly. Living in the present energizes what we do.

We don't eat the wrong things or overeat because we are hungry. We eat because it tastes good, now. It feels good in the mouth, now. It gives us pleasure, now.

And our brains remember that pleasure, prompting us to want to experience it again. When we first begin an exercise regimen we think of it as work. No matter how convinced we are of the need to work out on a regular basis, no matter how strong our belief in the need to prepare our body for the future, the time spent exercising can be difficult. We think of the exercise as effort. We are concentrating on getting that effort finished. It's not fun and our brains haven't clicked into pleasure. When just beginning an exercise program we may need to work on feeling enjoyment. After a time, when we have experienced pleasure because of some physical results, or experienced an endophin high, our brains will take care of the effort problem.

Athletes have fun. Who would scale a mountainside, or skydive, or play basketball if they disliked every minute of their activity? They are getting pleasure out of the moment. They are experiencing some satisfaction.

You want some of that. You don't necessarily want to do what they do; you just want to feel the good stuff in what you do and discover ways to enjoy the moment. And you can get there. To quote from Steven Johnson's *Mind Wide Open*: "People don't get in shape simply because it's in their long-term interests. They get in shape because working out makes them feel good and their brains remember that feeling." This last idea is not speculation or anecdotal. Recent brain research proves it is true.

Finding The Pleasure
Sedentary 45 year-old people with expanding waists can't expect to jump into an exercise program looking for pleasure and expect to keep up with a healthy 20 year-old. They can't even expect to keep up with a healthy in-shape 65 year-old.

And it would not be too bright for a sedentary person who has had an epiphany and feels the commitment to take off on a fast-paced long run. The dedication may be there, but it won't last long. If the sudden exertion doesn't shock the body into fatality, the strain and possible injury will drain away the dedication and enthusiasm.

You are not in this to hurt yourself. Working out, having fun, overdoing it and getting hurt, does little for your life. Finding enjoyment in exercise takes effort and balance, but it's worth it.

Active people who have shared their thoughts with me acknowledge that it is their thoughts and fantasies that help keep then on the exercise path.

What they do physically may not be what fits your body or may not include the exercises you choose to do. But our objective here is to use our minds, and I want to transfer some of what is in their heads into your head. I want to give you some tools to help in finding pleasure, and channeling your thoughts is an excellent tool.

A friend from the gym said he worked out because he constantly thinks of and enjoys the benefits. He said:

> "Seriously, I work out for four reasons. It
> literally keeps me sane. It clears and settles
> my mind and calms me. It grounds me in my
> body and gives me great endorphins. It's one
> of my best creative times — I can get on a
> machine with an idea, a problem or a project
> and I can work for an hour or so and get lots

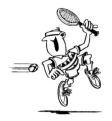

Our goals must be realistic. We are creatures of the moment. Living in the present energizes what we do. and can help us exercise regularly.

of great ideas. And finally, I have plans to live to about 108 years old, and I know that I need to have a good vehicle to have fun in, to play in, to do my life's work from and to enjoy all the gifts that life has to offer. If I want to make 108, I've got to really keep the thing healthy and tuned up."

Mary, who rides a stationary bike and uses weight machines in a fitness center, says her mind carries her off into sexual fantasies. In her own words:

"I exercise because I want to get naked and not be overcome with shame. I wish I could say it's because I want to be healthy but the truth is I mainly want to be attractive. Also, if I squat down I want to be able to get back up without looking for a chair back to grab on to. I want to go up a flight of stairs and not hear my own panting. I like it when I'm more agile. I've gone through a bunch of exercise phases: hefting free weights, hiking uphill, dancing like Michael Jackson, taking kayak lessons, imitating Madonna, riding the stationary bicycle, running on a treadmill and right now, playing racquetball. One thing I have learned from all of this is to give up my pride in how I look when I am exercising. I listen to audio tapes. Right now I'm listening to Joseph Campbell's *Varieties of Religious Experience*, Volume III. Last week I listened to Proust."

She came to her lifestyle of regular workouts, about age 45, along with a change of job and location. She realized that it would be necessary to improve her physical shape if she were to find and keep a new relationship. She wasn't looking for a model's body, just improved strength and flexibility. And that goal is essential for anyone who knows that a sexual, warm relationship is what they want from life.

Celina tells me she has started swimming again after being away from it for 10 years. She was a competitive swimmer during her teen years, then she stopped. She says:

> "I not only am enjoying the feel of my body
> during and after swimming, I am shocked
> at the memories that have awakened about
> those years. All the while I am swimming new
> remembrances come alive. It's like watching a
> movie and I just want to keep going."

Focusing only on the details of exercise can make the time appear to go on forever. If an exercise time frame becomes something you must do and get over with, it turns it into a task. Obligatory tasks aren't much fun. Thoughts and fantasies distract us, making the time go quickly.

Having creative fantasies while riding a stationary bike is fun for me. It wouldn't work if I were riding a bicycle in traffic, taking a step aerobics class, or competing in a sport where concentration on the task at hand is necessary.

At times, when preparing for a workshop or presentation, I start thinking about what I plan to talk about, mulling it over and over until I come up with a hook — sometimes two hooks — to hang the talk around. Over several days I build an outline around the hook, then start filling in the outline — all in my head — on the bike. I mull it over and over, then give the talk without writing anything down.

This technique took years to perfect, and I'm using it as an example of where a mind can go once exercise becomes a habit. The process is not only a distraction from the task at hand, it's satisfying.

My requirements, when I am exercising are to make it both fun and funny.

As an example: Kegels are exercises that women can do to sustain pelvic muscular strength. The literature says to pretend to hold back urine by contracting vaginal muscles, release and contract, release and contract. But that's not fun.

Instead, I pretend to swallow with my vagina. And I keep doing it. I listen to music when doing abdominal crunches. I get going to the music with the crunches, then I start the vaginal swallowing in rhythm.

Another time for "swallowing with your vagina" can happen when you are waiting in a grocery store checkout line. The magazines around the check stand could be a trigger, and it's great fun to put a little smile on your face because no one else knows what you are doing.

Kegel exercises do more than help keep you sexually able, they help in keeping you continent as you age. Those muscles need work. And before the males in the crowd start thinking this is funny, that flexing of those muscles helps keep prostrates healthy and prevents hemorrhoids. You may as well have fun, whether riding a stationary bike or doing Kegels.

Sometimes I only listen to music on a headset. Some trainers caution beginners not to use music while they exercise. On the other hand, some of the latest

38

research indicates we increase the physical benefits if we can work out while listening music we like.

If you are concerned about your hearing, use headphones with the little knobs, not ones that cover the whole inside of your ears. Then put the knobs a bit away from the ear canal. They can even be behind your ears resonating against your skull. That's probably the way Beethovan heard his music as his hearing was fading. I have my hearing checked every two years to make sure I maintain the same hearing level because I do listen to music quite a lot with headphones.

The main function of music for my husband David is to drive the pace of his time riding the exercise bike. When he is ready to sprint, fast music, combined with the adrenaline he feels coursing through his body, drives him through the vigor of the sprint. He says the time literally flies away.

Some exercise perfectionists are contemptuous of those who read while on a treadmill or bike. That too is nonsense. If reading, watching television, or listening to book tapes during your aerobics gets your heart rate up and keeps it up for at least 20 minutes, go for it. Whatever distracts, amuses, satisfies or turns you on is what works on the path to regular exercise. No one formula fits all. So consider the limitations of your own body, experiment with all available options, start slowly, and tell yourself it will become fun. Soon you'll reach your goal.

Your first goal is to make physical exercise pleasurable. Your second goal must be habit.

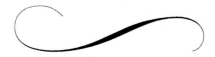

I've had people tell me that they exercise because they "have to." But they "hate" it. Hating something will beat out "have to" any day of the week. A part of developing physical consciousness is finding things to do that are pleasurable. It may take some talking to ourselves to get there. But get there we must. Without the pleasure a healthy lifestyle habit won't happen.

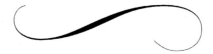

5 *Make Habit Your Friend*

A NECESSARY GOAL — HABIT. It can be your friend or your enemy.

We don't get up in the morning whining and complaining about brushing our teeth. We don't say : "I don't want to brush," or "I don't feel like it today, I'll do it tomorrow." If we are like 95% of the population, we just do it. If we forget to brush, our fuzzy mouths bother us all day.

Driving our car is a habit. When we were first learning we were acutely aware of every move, the feel and turn of the steering wheel, the gas pedal. After awhile we just did it. We don't stew about not wanting to drive. We don't fret about doing it right. We get in our cars, watch the traffic, and drive. We have acquired the habit. I know a 94 year-old who makes a habit of leaving her house every day, just so she'll keep moving!

We are creatures of pleasure and we are creatures of habit. So much of what we do daily, we do on automatic pilot. Our brains and bodies automatically send many routine chores into to a lower level of consciousness, setting up habits. Habits can be helpful tools. Bad habits can lead us to ill health and even early death.

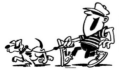 *Habits can be helpful tools. Bad habits can lead us to ill health and even early death.*

41

We are such creatures of habit that, for some, having to stray from a regular routine is upsetting. Go into any college classroom. When semesters begin most students pick a seat and go to that place during every subsequent class. Teachers advise college students to be sure to sit in their same seats when they take their final tests. Their seat is familiar, they need not waste mental energy and time adjusting to a different place, and they can concentrate on the test.

Another good example can be found in retirement homes. The residents choose to sit where they please in the dining room; but once they have chosen, they gravitate to that place every meal. In some cases, there can be a big fuss if someone else is sitting in their seat. The habit of "their" seat is comfortable. That's what they do.

Habit helps us get to work in the morning. Breaking a daily habit can make us late. Some people are rigidly tied to a regular schedule, so much so they come unglued if anything disrupts it. Less obsessive individuals can tolerate interruption and changes in a regular schedule, but habit is still useful in helping them accomplish what they want to get done.

Some of our habits easily fall into place. A three-year-old doesn't like brushing her teeth. But eventually she does it. Driving a car is complex, and it's a different kind of habit. We want it bad enough to cultivate it. Peer pressure comes into play — other people do it. We want to do it too. If they can do it, we can do it.

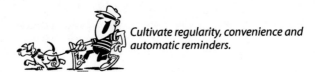

Cultivate regularity, convenience and automatic reminders.

Cultivating a habit

Like the driving habit, good lifestyle habits must be cultivated. If a bad-health epiphany gets you started, you must want a healthier body badly enough to cultivate the habit. If an aging epiphany gets you going; if a change in partners gets you going; if a lifestyle change gets you moving; whatever that light was that flashed in your head, it must be cultivated. It takes some persistence and regularity before the habit kicks in. If you experience some satisfaction from positive body changes the habit will kick in sooner. But the goal is habit, not body changes. Change will happen on its own.

The first principle of habit formation is regularity. Whatever you decide to do — whether it is to work out three times a week, or daily — decide on the time of day and hang onto that time as if your life depends on it. Even if you begin by disliking what you are doing, hang on to that time. The displeasure will go away, some pleasure will emerge.

Over time, when you have sharpened your sensitivity to physical sensations, you will notice a difference in how you feel on the days you do not exercise. David, my husband, after several years of regular exercise, says he feels "saggy" when he misses a day or two of his daily exercise habit.

As we age, the results of gravity are more apparent. Flesh and bones counter gravity more readily when they are in good shape. A healthy twenty year old may not feel saggy after missing regular exercise days. Young flesh stays in shape easier than older flesh. So the earlier you get started, the sooner your improved shape will counter the effects of gravity.

If you are working out with a partner and the partner wants to skip regular times, resist — go on your own, in your scheduled time.

If your scheduled time is early in the morning and last night you stayed up late and are clinging to the bed, get up. Once you are moving you will feel better.

I exercise first thing in the morning, six days a week, no matter what. But I sometimes still awaken and I want to cling to the bed — it's warm and cozy. I know that once my feet start moving I will be in rhythm. But I also know that if I lay there I will regret skipping my workout. The morning exercise is my personal habit. It belongs to me. It's mine. I own it. It is what I do.

The second principle is convenience. If you intend to use a fitness center, it must be readily accessible. You aren't likely to drive across town on a stormy day. Video tapes are convenient, living close to walking paths is convenient, having a "good" stationary bike is convenient. It's easier to build a habit around convenience.

A third principle is to build in automatic reminders. For mothers with young children, the time habit will be more difficult. This is a place to build in triggers or prompts. Children's nap time can be a trigger to do some exercise. While watching TV, the commercial break is a prompt to exercise. Do you know a friend with young children who wants to exercise? Trade child sitting. Raising children may not allow for a rigid schedule, so adapt to a more flexible habit. Flexibility takes more creativity and concentration. But if your epiphany is earth-shaking enough, you will find a way to establish that habit.

A rule of thumb about habit is: The first three days are the hardest. Recall learning to drive. After seven days habit building becomes easier. Then after fifteen days the habit begins to take hold. Head for fifteen days and keep going into mindless exercise habits. It's what you can do.

Once the habit is in place and is ingrained into your psyche, you may feel like making a fuss when the habit is interrupted, just like old people in retirement centers who can't sit in their same chair. They need that particular chair. You need that particular habit.

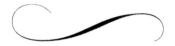

We are creatures of pleasure and we are creatures of habit. So much of what we do daily, we do on automatic pilot. Our brains and bodies automatically send many routine chores into to a lower level of consciousness, setting up habits. Habits can be helpful tools. Bad habits can lead us to ill health and even early death.

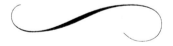

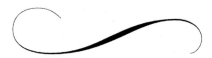

Most everything we do all day is habit. We can't think in getting rid of bad habits, we have to think in terms of developing new ones. It takes consciousness, talking to ourselves and work. Again to quote Dr. Richard Restak, "You do the fitness often enough and something marvelous happens. You and the fitness become one. Then the fitness does you." That's the habit kicking in.

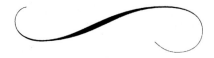

6 Designing Mind Games

OUR MINDS ARE NEVER STILL. We experience an internal constant dialogue, even while meditating. That running dialogue can keep us awake at night. It can keep us amused. It keeps us focused on a project. It helps us resolve problems. It keeps us in love or in hate.

If you have experienced the epiphany and developed some goals keep talking to yourself. Begin paying attention to what you are saying and thinking.

Self Talk

I often hear excuses when it comes to exercise. "I hate to exercise." "I know I should but I don't have the time."

"I guess I should, I'll do it someday." That's true enough. Physical therapists work in nursing homes helping residents keep their hips, knees, shoulders and other joints limber. Research programs in nursing homes demonstrate how arthritic joints can be improved with movement exercises. My advice for the "I'll get into exercise someday" game is to wait for the nursing home staff to help you. They can show you how to stretch your joints. Your choice.

I work in my garden that's enough" is another excuse. It's not enough. Gardening work is more like nursing home work where employees use their same muscles over and over, using some, neglecting others.

47

Gardening produces little opportunity to work on muscle balance, and little aerobic exercise at all.

"I hate it." My husband's mother used to say: "Mustn't hate." I say: "I can if I want to." You can if you want to, too. But if you hate exercise you may never get your body moving toward some life changes. The person you are would be trapped in a carrying case that can't move well. It may well hurt when you move, and you would need to hire someone to cut your toenails. Your choice.

Start a mantra, "I will learn to enjoy exercise." "I love exercise." That's not fibbing; it's self talk intended to assist in changing your anti-exercise processing.

If you are exercising regularly, begin to pay closer attention to your body changes. Notice a muscle that's a little larger: what a wonderful thing. Admire it; pat yourself on the back.

My Self Talk

My muscle building began in earnest when I was teaching a fitness class at a small gym. I had to thread my way through the big, black, heavy weight machines to get to the studio. Those machines were ominous. I decided to conquer them.

Starting slowly, I gradually went from machine to machine to learn which muscles each one strengthened. I would wear a head set and listen to music, then mentally run the music through the muscle I was strengthening while talking to the machine.

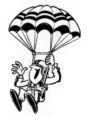

Start a mantra, "I will learn to enjoy exercise." "I love exercise." That's not fibbing; it's self talk intended to assist in changing your anti-exercise processing.

48

Then I read in a bodybuilding magazine about a small study indicating that when body builders talked to their muscles as they worked them, the muscles seemed to enlarge faster. So I began talking to my muscles. The talk may not have increased the size of my muscles, but the routine became fun. I most especially talk to my left bicep because it seems not to be able to grow as large as my right bicep.

A few months after I had begun using the weight machines I felt a lump on my side as I was leaving the gym. It was a newly found arm muscle, grown large enough to touch my side. What a deal! I patted myself on the back for that one.

I do not come from athletic people and will never have anything but a square, soft, endomorph body. But my muscles are strong and I admire them, talk to them, and enjoy them.

It is highly satisfying to walk up to a weight machine after some big guy has been using it, add some weight, and pull without scrinching my face. Part of not scrinching my face is habit. I'm well aware of how easily expressions can be etched into our faces so I concentrate on relaxing my face muscles when using weights.

Many exercises can do double duty. During my aerobics on a stationary bike, as I'm getting toward the end, I do a face lift. While still in a reverie I concentrate on the muscles in my face and pull them up. I am completely aware of this physical feeling. I saw a new face-lift procedure on television, where the doctor attached the cheek muscles to the bone under the eye. Ouch! So I do the same thing in my head. It seems much easier than the surgery. Six days a week I give myself a face lift for about three minutes.

I'm offering these personal mind games as examples of ways to use your ingenuity while exercising. It's easier to stay committed if you are enjoying some sense of the ridiculous.

My neighbor schedules fast walking with a friend. She knows that if she has committed to a special time she won't back out. She schedules what she calls "walk & talk" times with friends. They used to get together for coffee and eat and talk. Now she will go to a friend's house, walk in, and say: "lets go." They walk through a wooded park for two hours, enjoy a great visit and then she goes home. No stopping for coffee and eating.

She said she had one friend who could only go in the early mornings. So for one year they walked and talked in the dark early morning, many times in the rain. She never would have felt comfortable walking alone at that hour, but with the two of them, they felt safe.

Here are some thoughts from a 65 year old man who exercises in a swimming pool to exercise and soothe his rheumatoid-arthritic joints:

"I used to golf and play tennis, but I couldn't do
either anymore so I had to find alternatives.
I knew exercise was good for me and I felt
better when I could. Three times a week I
swim laps in the municipal pool for pain relief
and to improve my respiration. In addition, I
do some stretching exercises in the pool. I like
to swim and I enjoy the guys and gals I swim

50

with. Then I go twice a week to a center for therapy. A lot of people there to interact with. More conversation there. It's become part of my life. Sometimes while I'm swimming laps I problem-solve. Other times I work on a poem. There are some attractive women there, so sometimes I fantasize."

He problem-solves, as do many people when they are working out. He fantasizes. He uses his exercise time as a social get together. Socialization during exercise workouts is an excellent pleasure goal if the time is available. He didn't elaborate on his fantasies as some of my interviewees have. But fantasies can be amazing pleasurable distractions while improving cardiac capability.

I'll offer another game. The stationary bikes I use are equipped with heart sensors, so off and on I measure my heart rate just to note where I am and to play a game. I start slowly, build up, go fast for about twenty minutes, then cool down. I know that the healthier the heart, the easier it is for the pulse rate to drop. When I'm about finished I reduce the resistance level to low, pedal slowly and watch my heart rate slow down. My goal is at least a 30 beat drop within a minute — for example, from a rate of 150 to under 115.

I suspect that biofeedback is part of what I do when lowering my heart rate on the exercise bike. Once I tried slowing my pulse rate to demonstrate that possibility and I frightened my husband. The look on his face was pure astonishment.

Triggers

Triggers are events, personal encounters or opportunities that remind you to do a specific exercise, such as standing up straight, tightening your gut, stretching, or going into a favorite fantasy. Grocery store checkout lines provide an opportunity for my favorite exercise of tightening my pelvic muscles. Another prompt is stairs or curbs, which help me tighten my abdominal muscles. Watching hunched over bodies in nursing homes helps improve my posture. I stride out of a nursing home, thoroughly appreciating my leg and abdominal muscles.

You can design your own triggers. An irritating person you encounter several times a day could offer a prompt to stand straight and tense your gut. A set of stairs can provide an opportunity to stretch your legs. A television commercial offers time to stand and stretch. These little things add up to a lot of physical benefit over a lifetime.

An Emotional Tool

Another little surprise you might encounter is an endorphin hit. Endorphins are neurotransmitters released from the brain into the body that reduce pain and make us feel good.

I recall sedentary people commenting on how difficult it must be for joggers because their faces look so hot and sweaty when they finish. Running may be

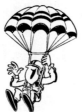

Triggers are events, personal encounters or opportunities that remind you to do a specific exercise, such as standing up straight, tightening your gut, stretching, or going into a favorite fantasy.

difficult for anyone who dislikes jogging and is only doing it to get the exercise, but most runners who enjoy the sport will admit that no matter how hot and sweaty their faces are, they feel great at the end of a run. That high after a workout is a reward.

Ample evidence demonstrates the benefits of regular exercise on depression. One of my sons was going through a divorce, and he was deeply depressed. I added him onto my fitness center membership so he could work out. He says to this day, that having that gym membership saved his life.

Scientific conclusions are still out on whether it is positive or negative to use exercise to vent anger or frustration. But I had a personal therapeutic payoff in using exercise to deal with anger that was eating into my days. I would physically punch at the imaginary object of my distress while doing aerobics in my living room. I would kick in the direction of where the person lived. Step on his imaginary head, jump so hard I visualized blood flowing. Soon I noticed that the only time I was disturbed was while doing the exercise. My days were becoming free of distress. Then one day I noticed I was punching at a different injustice — I was home free. This exercise stuff does a lot more than just build strong bodies; it is a tool for changing our emotions.

Use anything you can think of to propel you to get started and stay with it. Use your mind to take you into another realm: For some it may be prayer; for others daydreams, Some will find sexual fantasies and power fantasies. Music tapes, book tapes, and reading help while doing aerobics. Work out with your friends. You can find new friends to exercise with.

53

And opportunities present themselves frequently: Fitness classes, fitness trainers, fitness centers, dance classes, movement classes, running, jogging, fast walking, tennis, swimming, real bikes, stationary bikes, treadmills. You can buy or rent exercise videos with beautiful people and you can watch similar classes on cable television. You can do simple things like exercising with stretch bands. You can enroll in step classes or yoga classes. You can use exercise to enjoy life now and use the benefits of exercise to enjoy life later. Talk to yourself about that idea.

There are no guarantees for our later years. Our life satisfaction depends on genetics, luck, and the choices we have made. We would regret, however, having won out on genetics and luck and then blowing it with poor lifestyle choices.

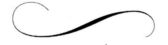

We have a constant dialogue going on in our heads all the time. Developing a consciousness about that dialogue and channeling it into lifestyle change will help keep us on the straight and narrow.

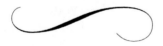

7 *Aerobics*

THE OPTIMUM REQUIREMENTS FOR PHYSICAL health are aerobics, some strength building and some stretching. Aerobics can be anything from fast walking to running to bicycling, as long as it's a steady stretch of time — preferably at least 20 minutes.

Aerobic exercises are rhythmic, use the major muscle groups and are sustained at a continuous intensity. Because both the cardiovascular and respiratory systems come into play, continued aerobic exercise benefits blood vessels and lungs as well as the heart. Health aside, all that oxygen-rich blood flowing easily through our bodies pumps up the skin and improves our looks.

However, people are often confused about aerobic exercise. Just because you're breathing hard and your heart is pumping does not necessarily mean you are giving your heart the exercise it needs to improve long-term cardiac health.

Our bodies use energy in two basic processes: Anaerobic — working without depending on oxygen for energy; and Aerobic — using an oxygen-rich system for energy.

Anaerobic provides a quick burst of energy output. For example, suppose you suddenly see a child about to tumble off a porch and you quickly jump and save the child from falling. The energy that enabled your muscles to move that quickly lies in a two part chemical system within the muscles. You don't have enough time to generate the oxygen needed for fuel so the first chemical system — phosphagen — provides energy for approximately 20 seconds to 1 minute. When that is used up the second chemical — lactic acid — kicks in and fuels the muscles for up to 3 minutes. By that time, if you continue moving quickly, you are breathing hard and oxygen is fueling those muscles.

Playing basketball, with its quick starts and stops is using the anaerobic system. Lifting weights for muscle building or any sport that requires a spurt of effort for a few minutes, then a pause, is anaerobic.

Breathing hard after a quick burst isn't aerobic exercise, it's a recovery time to replenish our anaerobic chemical energy system. It's complicated, but hey, we are complicated beings.

During the day, most of our energetic needs are provided by the aerobic system. When significant muscular effort is required — like climbing stairs or lifting a heavy object — then our bodies briefly engage the chemical energy (anaerobic) system.

When I jump on a stationary bike and start pedaling fast, for the first three minutes my muscles are depending on the chemical energy system. Then the remaining time on my bike would be using the steady aerobic system.

It's that steady aerobic exercise over a 20 to 30 minute time that builds the heart's stamina so it will be able to pump more oxygenated blood with less effort, making the whole system work better. It builds the heart's capability to increase its stroke volume, or the amount of oxygenated blood moved with every beat. Then the heart doesn't need to work so hard to supply the body. If the stroke volume (or amount of oxygenated blood) the heart pushes out with every beat is small and our extremities require more oxygen for the energy we are expending, then the heart must pump much faster — it's working under stress.

Depending on our stamina and state of health, aerobic exercise can be anything sustained, such as walking, jogging, stair climbing or jumping rope.

Some evidence indicates that if exercise time is limited, aerobic exercise for 10 minutes three times a day benefits the heart. And if 10 minutes is all the time available, go for it. If it were me, I would try to stretch the time out whenever possible for at least 13 minutes to give my heart the full oxygen benefit of the 10 minutes.

And aerobic exercise encompasses so many things — from brisk walking, dancing, riding a bicycle — to taking aerobic fitness classes.

Of course anyone beginning an exercise program should be certain their heart is reasonably healthy. And those with damaged hearts must start slowly and gradually increase under the guidance of a professional. I repeat: We are in this to be healthy, not hurt ourselves.

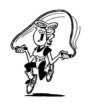

It is possible to change how you feel by changing how your body moves.

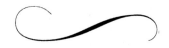

Because both the cardiovascular and respiratory systems come into play, continued aerobic exercise benefits blood vessels and lungs as well as the heart. Health aside, all that oxygen-rich blood flowing easily through our bodies pumps up the skin and improves our looks.

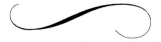

8 *Muscles*

OUR MUSCLES ARE SUCH AN IMPORTANT PART of a dynamic living system, yet we tend to ignore them until something goes wrong. But muscle building need not include buffing up, oiling down, and standing on a stage flexing. Yet the thought of having to push and strain like body builders is what keeps many of us away from strength building as well as keeping us from the enormous benefits strong muscles provide.

The Benefits

If our leg muscles are reasonably strong they complement the cardiac system. Strong legs are sometime referred to as a second heart. They aid the heart by pushing the de-oxygenated blood back up through our bodies to get fresh oxygen from our lungs and keep us fit.

Think about it: First, there's lots of blood in the legs. Second, that blood is farthest from the heart. Third, that blood, being closer to the ground, is more strongly pulled by gravity away from the heart."

Strong muscles also help keep calcium in bones. Tendons connect our muscles to our bones. Restrict movement and let muscles go soft and we will lose calcium, literally urinating out more calcium than we take in. Bones become porous and thin, leading to the dreaded osteoporosis.

Developed muscles burn calories all the time, even while we sleep, improving our metabolism. Strong

59

muscles require those calories just to exist. Stop working a muscle and it shrinks. Flesh without much muscle just lays there inert. A good example is the appearance of a healed broken limb when it is removed from the cast. The muscle appears to have disappeared.

But even if you believe in the value of developed muscles, where is the fun in working on them if you dislike fitness centers and hate the thought of lifting weights?

The options to help you are diverse. Exploring those options requires some creative thinking and a little bit of experimentation. Video tapes and cable television offers many exercise programs. Tape TV programs so you can exercise at convenient times.

Read muscle magazines on how to use weights correctly. Those magazines are expensive, but can be helpful. I read them while waiting in a grocery store line (along with flexing my vaginal muscles), and have learned more about correct ways of strengthening my muscles with weights and machines then I ever did with instruction from a trainer.

You need not invest in expensive equipment. For beginners, the weight need not be terribly heavy. Small weights are sold in variety stores. Cans of food can work well in a pinch. If you start feeling successful and find a muscle or two getting larger, you just might want to explore using heavier weights.

"What a crime it is for a man to grow old without knowing the strength and beauty of which his body is capable."
— Socrates

60

Muscle Balancing

But no matter what weights you use, a lifestyle of exercise requires muscle balancing. Muscles are wonderfully powerful and demand the right to be treated with care. Strengthening a muscle on one side also requires the opposing muscle to be strengthened. Those working in physically challenging occupations will claim they need no extra exercise because they use their muscles enough. But using the same muscles over and over with only a few muscles getting the workout can cause problems.

For example, nursing home employees lift and strain many times during the day. Strength may build in arm muscles for a while, but in so many cases the opposing muscles are getting little or nothing. Using back muscles alone without strengthening stomach muscles makes that occupation one of the most hazardous for back injuries.

A case in point: I knew a young man who had lost an arm when he was ten years old. He had decided he could play baseball with one arm as well as anyone with two arms, and he played. Around age 15 someone finally noticed that his body looked rather strange. He had developed the muscles on one side of his body, while neglecting the muscles on the other side. The strong muscles had twisted his spine around so that the weak side of his rib cage was in front of his body. He lived in a body cast for a year in an attempt to straighten his spine, but he has never reached a balance in his posture.

The way to think of muscle balance is: front of the body versus back of the body; side of the body versus the other side of the body. Or at a smaller level: front of the arm versus back of the arm; side of the arm versus other side of the arm.

Pay attention to what muscles you use when working or playing and practice flexing them to build strength. You can learn to use the things you do daily to keep balanced.

The funny kegel exercises to strengthen pelvic muscles are a serious matter. Continency for older women can become a life-controlling issue. A client I worked with had "made it" in terms of what we can hope for towards the end of our lives. She was 92 years old, living alone in her own home, quite capable of using the stairs. Her mind was sound, she had many friends of all ages, and her family cared dearly for her. She had made it until her developing bladder problems sent her off to her doctor, who handed her a box of latex gloves and advised her that when her bladder started poking out through her vagina, to just put on a glove and push it back up. The thought horrifies me. It horrified that woman so much that she refused to leave her home. She would not allow her bladder to become full. She went downhill from there with a life that could only focus on staying put, near a bathroom.

Bladders tend to drop over time because gravity works well when the supporting muscles begin to atrophy. Her sad story certainly made me get in touch with my Kegel exercises. But I went from sad and determined to having fun with thinking I am funny when doing abdominal crunches or standing in a grocery store line.

Leg muscles will improve with aerobics — walking, running, bicycling, tennis, playing running games, step classes — you can discover so many options. The more variety you incorporate in your life, the more balanced the leg muscles.

The Magic Muscle

I want to emphasize one set of muscles that bears special consideration and attention because those muscles can affect our lives so profoundly. Pay close attention to your abdominal muscles. Those muscles are not only magical and powerful, they are crucial to your overall health.

Most of us know that if abdominal muscles are strong, the back is supported and we are less likely to suffer lower back pain. However, behind the lower abdominal muscles are our intestines. That's where nutrients from our food are absorbed and where the waste is eliminated. If stomach muscles sag, the intestines sag and become less efficient. If older adults' intestines sag they tend to not get all the nutrients from what they eat and have difficulty with elimination.

Rising above the intestines is the stomach. When abdominal muscles sag, intestines sag, and the stomach sags. When food hits a sagging stomach it doesn't start to digest easily, leading to hiatal hernia and acid reflux that we call heartburn.

If our abdominal muscles are strong and hold our intestines and stomach up in place, our lungs stay up.

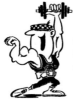

Gender aside, a strong capable body is beautiful at any age.

If our lungs are up in place we aerate better, making it easier for our hearts to pump that oxygenated blood through our bodies. The better our blood flow, the nicer our skin and the smarter our brain. How's that for a hard sell?

More important, achieving strong abdomen muscles does not require a thousand sit ups a day. In fact, those popular sit ups are not an efficient way to work those muscles, and such exercises can hurt your back muscles and spine.

Abdominal crunch exercises work if they are done right. Lay on your back. Bend your knees, put your feet on the floor lined up about shoulder width. If you are a person who has already done crunches, do them your way. Now do them my way. Push the small of your back into the floor. Not just a little — a lot. My dance instructor once said, "If I walked up and acted like I would stomp you in the gut, you would push into the floor. That's how hard to push that back to the floor." She would say, "Crack a walnut with the small of your back." She would say, "Pretend the door to Pandora's box is at the small of your back. If you let up at all, all the furies in the netherland will invade the world. It's up to you to save the world. Hold that door shut with all of your might."

Now do little crunches. The secret is how hard the small of the back is pushed into the floor. Do crunches until you feel those abdominal muscles. Do crunches in rhythm to music. If you are a woman, get the rhythm going and start moving the vaginal muscles to improve circulation, hold the bladder in place and help keep you sexually able. If you are male, flex the rectal and lower pelvic muscles. Remember, it's good for the prostate and can prevent hemorrhoids, too.

Here's an even more effective abdominal exercise (the secret to this exercise is in the breathing):

Stand, feet slightly apart. Lean your weight a little forward on the balls of your feet, but keep your heels on the floor. Stand tall, feel yourself being straight. Now breathe normally. Keep breathing in a regular rhythm, do not stop. Clench those gut muscles like a fist. Practice that a lot. When you get really good at it and can feel the clench, mentally attach the clenched muscle to your back. Keep breathing normally in a regular rhythm.

Now, you can get all dressed up, stand in front of a mirror, breathe as before, clench the gut muscles, pull them toward your back, and walk away from the mirror, still breathing and holding the stomach in. You can go to the party, walk through the door and keep your stomach held up.

A word of caution: Most of us get all dressed up, stand in front of the mirror, hold our breath and suck in our guts. Lovely. Except, that gut is held in with some mighty powerful muscles. Right when our heart needs the oxygen to attempt to feed those muscles, we are holding our breath. Fortunately, nature takes over as we step away, we breathe, and our stomachs pop out. That's probably just fine for women, but not too good for overweight men. Women tend to form most of their fat on the outside of their abdominal muscles. Men form fat behind those muscles. Ever hear some man with a large gut say: "Feel how hard my stomach is?" That's because he can flex that muscle in front of his fat. So if his heart isn't in good shape and he holds his breath and sucks his stomach in, he can kill himself. He not only is denying powerful muscles the oxygen they need, he is pushing fat back against his insides and against his heart.

I try not to teach this exercise to overweight males until they understand the danger of holding their breath and sucking in. For all of you, keep breathing: those powerful abdominal muscles really need the heart to keep pumping oxygen through the blood. The heart is strained if you are not breathing.

If it's really important to you, you will practice breathing and clenching those muscles, then build in visual triggers or prompts to tighten the gut. I breathe, clench, and suck in when I go up stairs, or up a sidewalk curb. I do this tightening while waiting in grocery store lines also. We all must find our own triggers for a specific exercise, but a little habit with this exercise produces great benefits.

We can feel and look better than our peers when we are 90 years old, because our midsections will not sag, keeping our intestines in place so we can absorb the nutrients from our food. We won't experience bathroom problems. Our esophaguses will not drop down into our stomachs, and we'll avoid acid reflux.

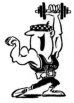

Developed muscles burn calories all the time, even while we we sleep, improving our metabolism. Strong muscles require those calories just to exist. Stop working a muscle and it shrinks. Flesh without much muscle just lays there inert. A good example is the appearance of a healed broken limb when it is removed from the cast. The muscle appears to have disappeared.

Our lungs will aerate better, our hearts will pump easier, and our brains will be quicker.

A word of caution however, for anyone with much excess weight on them. Gravity works, and jogging, running, jumping rope all feed into gravity's pull on bouncing flesh. Whatever exercise you are doing attempt to avoid that bouncing. It is especially important for abdomens, which can become saggy from the bouncing. Even those without extra flesh should consider some support for that stomach area when running.

Ordinarily I am critical of the big promises made by fitness instructors and trainers when we are promised great beauty from exercise. But with the work on abdominal muscles, I make one mighty big promise that is better than mere beauty. Strengthen those muscles in the stomach area and a whole lot of life will function easier than your friends whose stomachs hang low.

To quote Socrates: "What a crime it is for a man to grow old without knowing the strength and beauty of which his body is capable." Gender aside, a strong capable body is beautiful at any age.

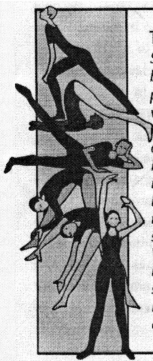

The knee bone's connected ...

Strong pelvic muscles help hold our bladders in place, prevent lower back pain and keep our guts from sagging so we look better. When our guts sag our intestines droop, causing less efficient digestion and elimination. When our intestines sag our stomach riding above it sags, leading to discomfort, hiatal hernias and heartburn, which frequently occur in people with weak stomach muscles and poor posture. When our stomach droops the lungs riding above it sag. If our lungs don't sag we aerate more efficiently making it easier on our hearts and getting more oxygen to the brain.

9 *Flexibility*

THE BETTER OUR RANGE OF MOTION, the smoother we walk through life. There is a world of difference in how society perceives older adults who walk firmly, strongly, with smooth strides compared to those older adults who shuffle along. Nature set us up so we are attracted to stronger bodies.

A strong, vital adult is treated differently than a frail, dependent adult because at some level we understand the latter require attentive care. So we speak to them as we speak to children who need that care. Sometimes we tend to not even engage frail people in an adult conversation. I do not want to be spoken to as if I were a dependent child. And I want to be free to move about with ease.

Research demonstrates that even extremely frail nursing home residents have built strength and improved flexibility with exercise. If these frail, old bodies can become more flexible and so can ours, provided we use our unique individuality and choose our expectations realistically.

We can keep that healthy range of motion and those smooth-moving joints by extending the joints to their full range on a regular basis with exercise.

The better our range of motion, the smoother we walk through life.

Our joints contain a fluid — synovial fluid — that is necessary to keep them moving or rotating or whatever else they do. The larger the range of motion in a joint, the more synovial fluid is available to the joint. The tighter the joint has become, the less fluid is available and the more likely the joint will stiffen.

Gravity will really do a number on us if we don't stay stretched. As we age our collagen cells shrink. Collagen dominates all of our connective tissue: our skin, our ligaments, our tendons; there is even a bit of collagen in our bones.

For some reason, maybe because of gravity, the collagen in our lower body tightens more quickly than in our upper body. If an older woman who has not stayed flexible falls or wrenches a hip in the wrong direction, the skin and ligaments do not give. Instead, the bone gives. Even those experiencing slight bone loss can break a hip because of this phenomena. And the tightening can happen in short time.

For example, suppose an older woman maintains a large home. She goes up and down stairs; she works in her yard; she reaches into cupboards. All normal routines. She then decides to make life easier, selling her home and moving into a much smaller apartment in a retirement community.

At first she is a bit depressed about the move and stays in her smaller home adjusting to the newness and slowly adapting. She starts becoming social again and noticing how much more difficult it is to move about, thinking that perhaps the move was a good thing because her body is becoming stiff.

However, her body didn't just begin stiffening because of age; it stiffened because the moving about required in her larger home has stopped.

I'm not advocating that older people keep their large homes forever. In fact, the more moves we make, the more adaptable we become. I am advocating that should we move to smaller quarters we make sure we get the stretching exercise we need to keep moving.

Stretching does not require a special time. It can be done periodically during the day, even while brushing your teeth. Now that we are aware of our teeth-brushing habit we can enlarge upon it by incorporating hip rotations. Start brushing, plant your feet shoulder-length apart and circle those hips in rhythm with the brushing. You might not want to do it if the bathroom door is open and there are guests in the house.

Developing a stretching habit requires regularity and common sense. Yoga classes are excellent places if the instructor is instructing and not showing off. In class situations we tend to follow instructions so we won't stand out from the rest of the class. That conformity can push us beyond what we are capable of doing.

I recently attended a yoga class where the teacher was demonstrating his prowess and asked everybody, even newcomers, to do the plow. That's an exercise where you lay on your back, raise your hips and put your feet on the floor behind your head. The latest advice on the plow is: Don't do it. It's harmful to upper backs and necks. Even if the instructor was unaware of the

Nature set us up so we are attracted to stronger bodies.

ban on the plow, he should have cautioned newcomers and demonstrated alternative stretches.

However, really good yoga classes not only provide demonstration for slow joint stretching, they are good for getting in touch with our unique selves that live in our carrying cases. Yoga teaches us to focus.

But not everyone can get to a class. In that case, the video tapes and good books on stretching and yoga are easily available from bookstores and libraries.

Stretching before aerobic exercise should be brief — five seconds at the most — and not too vigorous, for each stretch. Joints are cold when we begin and the stretching is designed to gently warm them up. After aerobic exercise joints should be stretched and the stretch position held for at least 20 seconds. These stretches help increase the range of motion because the joints are warm.

We can stretch in bed in the morning before we get up. Watch a cat awaken from a nap and notice the gentle stretches. We can stretch while we are getting dressed. We can stretch and move several times during the day when we are working. An added benefit of stretching while working at a sedentary job is that it reduces fatigue, improves breathing and reduces the chances of injury from repetitive motion tasks.

I keep a pole in my office and use it to rotate my shoulders after being on the computer for hours. I keep a stretch cord there also because my back appreciates a stretch or two during the day.

Stretching and flexing while watching television, especially during the commercials, counteracts all the work the couch is doing to force our bodies into the shape of a potato.

Before going to bed, stretching and flexing helps to prevent joint and muscle aches that can develop while we sleep. We can get up and stretch during the night if our backs hurt.

If you are a beginner and new to exercise, begin slowly and carefully. If you need inspiration, sit on a park bench and the watch the differences in how bodies move. Look for younger people who move as if they had 90 years on them. Look for gray heads that move with ease. Look for everything in between, then stand up, stretch your muscles, rotate your shoulders, slightly arch and contract your spine and pay attention to how you feel. If you have been made particularly aware of a passerby or two whose bodies were shaped poorly and who walked with difficulty, say to yourself, "When I grow up I don't want to walk like that.

There is a world of difference in how society perceives older adults who walk firmly, strongly, with smooth strides compared to those older adults who shuffle along.

73

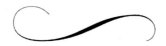

It is true. The greater our range of motion, the easier we walk through life. Too many older adults, who have no illness or disease, develop that old age shuffle. Staying flexible keeps our joints fluid.

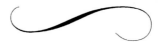

10 *The Brain*

"Keep learning. Learn more about the computer, crafts, gardening, whatever. Never let the brain idle. ' An idle mind is the devil's workshop.' And the devil's name is Alzheimer's."
— George Carlin

NOW WE KNOW: OUR BRAINS NOT ONLY NEVER LOSE the power to transform themselves on the basis of experience, they were constructed to change.

For decades conventional belief held that we were born with a given number of brain cells, were sloughing them off over a lifetime and could not generate new cells, nor could we activate new neural pathways. But recent scientific research about our brains has unearthed some dramatic results.

Neuroscientists have discovered that not only does the brain change throughout life, new neural stem brain cells can be generated in the hippocampus, a part of the brain that is vital for learning. We can generate and integrate new cells into existing brain circuits by engaging in new experiences and by practicing aerobic exercise.

Scientists are searching for the ways that gene therapy, drugs, or growth hormones might stimulate brain cell growth to counteract the many illnesses that can plague us. However, the consensus concludes that a change of lifestyle can stimulate brain growth in normal healthy people. Healthy brains can become "better" as physical activity and mental challenges provide natural stimulation.

75

How To Improve Your Brain

Our many levels of consciousness range from being fully alert and concentrating all the way down to barely functioning in a coma. As we are experiencing something new the brain is firing with lots of electrical activity. As we learn with concentration the task becomes easier, our brains fire less and less.

As an example, during a procedure called a functional magnetic resonance imaging (fMRI) a person's brain can be monitored while learning to play a piece of music without looking at the keyboard. Initially that brain is brightly firing reds and yellows As the task becomes easier and easier the brain fires less and less until there are just a few blues and greens.

Keeping the brain stimulated seems to be the important factor in keeping it healthy. To illustrate

fMRI (functional magnetic resonance imaging), uses radio waves and a strong magnetic field to measure the quick, tiny metabolic changes that take place in the active part of the brain. The fMRI. PET (positron emission tomography), EEG (electro-encephalogram, and MEG (magnetoencephalogram) allow researchers to record activity in the working brain and draw inferences about how the brain functions.
— F. Sommer & A. Wichert
    Exploratory Analysis &
    Data Modeling in Functional Neuroimaging.

this, suppose you are walking in your own familiar neighborhood. While you are walking, your body and your brain at some level of consciousness, know where you are. You are able to carry on a conversation, think many thoughts, hum a tune, make plans for another day. But if you were suddenly dropped down onto a street in Paris your brain would go on high alert. Live on that same street in Paris for a month and pretty soon the familiarity allows your brain to stop paying close attention and the walk on the street drops to a lower level of consciousness.

When we are initially learning a new skill or adapting to a new situation our brains are brightly firing. As the skill or the situation becomes old hat, our brains fire less and less as they adjust to the task.

Another example comes from the book *Aging With Grace* by David Snowdon, Ph.D. Dr. Snowdon reports research on nuns who have donated their brains to science. As they age, they are given yearly cognitive tests. When they die their brains are autopsied. The pathologist who does the autopsy then meets with the research team and in most cases has been able to tell where the person was on the cognitive tests by having examined the condition of their brain. Two nuns whose brains should have indicated severe dementia were exceptions They performed well on the cognitive tests up until their death even with brains littered with the dreaded plaques and tangles.

Dr. Snowden promised to keep the nuns fully informed on the research and he said he felt some chagrin when he told them that the stay-at-home sisters who cared for the convent were the ones whose brains deteriorated more quickly. Overall, the nuns who joined as young women and went on to teach and earn degrees seemed to maintain brain health well into old age.

The stay-at-home nuns were able to do their tasks without piquing their alert consciousness. The chores became rote. Their brains weren't required to fire with new information and tasks.

Another example comes from a study in Dr. Richard Restak's book, *Mozart's Brain & The Fighter Pilot*. Two students take a reasoning and intelligence test with their brains hitched to a Pet Scan. (See box on page 76.)

One brain shows lots of activity with an increase of red and oranges on a color-coded map. The other student's brain has far less activity with green and blues. Yet strange as it may seem, the student who scores the highest has the brain with less activity. The test was easier and he did not need to work so hard.

Our object then is to keep both brain and body alert, aware, and learning all the time. Both our brains and our bodies tend to want to maximize energy by adapting to new information then letting it slide into a level of consciousness that requires less effort. Much of the chronic ailments of older age afflict those who seem to be unaware of their own bodies. They don't pay attention until pain or illness strikes.

"You do the fitness often enough and something marvelous happens. You and the fitness become one. Finally, the fitness does you."
— Richard Restak, neurologist

78

Computer users can stimulate their brains by simply using their mouse with their other hand. Adjusting to the awkwardness and developing the skill to use the other hand requires the brain to get to work.

Going for a walk and dribbling a basketball with one hand, then switching to the other hand on the way back, fires the brain. It is a challenge and takes concentration.

Taking dance or step classes that require turning, balancing and learning new routines requires the old brain to really fire up and all the while we are so busy concentrating we don't even think about the aerobic benefits that are going on. It seems that just learning to balance on one foot is not only an exercise to prevent falls, it's a brain exercise.

And that brain/body connection works the other way also. One study measured a muscle in two groups of people and asked one group to concentrate on that muscle to make it stronger and bigger. When the groups were remeasured, the concentration group had increased muscle strength.

Early in this book I talked about my game of giving myself a face lift while riding a stationary bike and listening to music. I theorized I could concentrate on my face and make the muscle pull up and tighten. It may work. It may not work. But I have fun doing it. I think it's funny and the time goes by quickly during my aerobics. And I might well have had many more wrinkles and grooves if I hadn't been doing the imaginary face lifts. Now I have located some research to back up my theory. I've even found studies indicating that putting a smile on our faces when feeling down will lift our spirits.

79

Recent brain studies are producing amazing results. Some indicate that the brain in stroke victims can be forced to heal the body when the unaffected side is tied down, forcing the victim to use the damaged side of the body. The brain develops new pathways around the damage to force the weakened side to respond. For a brief time after a stroke the viable brain can regenerate new cells and pathways. What stimulates the regeneration is movement and use.

As my own fitness research project for over twenty years I do the brain games: Moving my computer mouse to the other side; dribbling a basketball; playing basketball; taking step classes; teaching jazz dance classes; testing to become certified for fitness training. And I believe I have experienced something that would not have been possible without those experiences. I can play the piano.

As a child in boarding school I took piano lessons from the fifth through eighth grades. I do not remember what I played. All I recall is: Biting a finger or two when they played a wrong note too many times; my mother being upset over having to purchase a formal dress for a recital; and teaching a younger child to play.

Then I did not touch a piano for 55 years. Recently my son brought his piano to store in my office and I

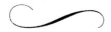

"The best ways to augment brain function might not involve drugs or cell implants, but lifestyle changes. Like many other organs, the brain responds positively to exercise, a good diet and adequate sleep."
— Fred Gage, *Brain, Repair Yourself*

decided to borrow some beginning books to relearn reading music. As I was practicing my husband brought home a Bach piece he especially liked. I told him it was much too difficult. Then, to my astonishment, I discovered I could play that Bach piece.

The experience encouraged me to purchase many more music books and within three months I could play rather complicated pieces, amazing my family and friends. As one son said, "who knew?" Then he said, "you could have taught us to play when we were kids." I wish I had had known to do that. Substantial evidence indicates the value of teaching children to read music.

It still feels strange. At times it's as if someone else is in my head and hands. What I had learned as a child came crashing out of my brain. It is a pleasant surprise and I am convinced that the brain exercises I have been doing allowed that to appear.

Fitness is more than a state of mind, it is a mind saver. And with the growing population of aging baby boomers, saving the mind as well as the body should become a priority. There will be so many older people in this country. If too many are frail and dependent the cost will be high in terms of providing care. It's up to us to take charge of our own aging.

I not only hope to be able to cut my own toenails until I leave this earth, I want to remember what my toes are.

Fitness is more than a state of mind, it is a mind saver. And with the growing population of aging baby boomers, saving the mind as well as the body should become a priority. There will be so many older people in this country. If too many are frail and dependent the cost will be high in terms of providing care. It's up to us to take charge of our own aging.

*The wonders of our brains have become my passion. Especially the new findings in the past 5 years. I heartily suggest reading Dr. Restak's **The New Brain and Mozart's Brain & The Fighter Pilot**. Talk about mind games.*

11 *Food*

WE DON'T OVEREAT BECAUSE WE'RE HUNGRY. We overeat because it tastes good and we are pleasure-oriented. And for some people food is an addiction. In fact, the areas of our brain that light up for cocaine are the same areas that light up when we overeat.

There is, however, a ray of hope coming from recent brain research where investigators demonstrated that our brains can be rewired to change our addictions. It's not easy and takes time, but with a lot of effort, talking to ourselves, and building new eating habits our brains will eventually stop jumping into cravings when we see something that is bad for the body, but good in the mouth. Advertisers understand the addiction. That's why pictures of hamburgers are flashed on television screens.

Changing eating habits is easier said than done. But it might be helpful if you understood that, over time, avoiding rich foods won't be painful. I was a child who would put brown sugar and powdered cocoa into a cup and hide it under my bed so I could eat it at night. Loved it.

For many years I found that avoiding rich things was a terrible hardship so I would yo-yo diet a lot. It wasn't until the exercise habit kicked in years ago, and I made an effort to eat for my health, that the addiction has gone.

A first step into healthy eating is paying attention to ourselves and what we eat. Eating is like all the other things we do during a day. It's a habit and lack of awareness

Once, when I was pouring sugar in my tea, a relative told me: "That's too much sugar. It's not good for you. I worry about you." At the same time that person had a big piece of chocolate cake in front of them. They didn't seem to understand the difference in relationship between putting sugar in tea and eating chocolate, butter, flour and sugar. My fasting blood sugar is tested once a year. It's 86. The recommended Diabetes Association guideline for normal is less than 110.

How I eat works for me but may seem strange to you. I don't eat breakfast first thing upon arising because I'm not hungry then. I drink half a cup of coffee with rice milk, then go to the gym. When I return home I grab a red yam, wash it, stab it a few times, wrap it in a paper towel and toss it into the microwave. While the yam cooks I stir-fry many vegetables. The freezer is full of frozen vegetables to use when fresh is not available. For my base I use spinach, cabbage, and tomatoes. I then add four or five other vegetables and the cooked yam, put a favorite sauce on top, and eat it. By that time I feel famished and it tastes so good. I read somewhere that yams are especially beneficial for women and that spinach is good for the eyes, so those vegetables are always part of the meal. Later in the day, when hunger creeps in, I throw frozen blueberries into a bowl; they are supposed to be good for the brain. I add sugar, uncooked quick-cooking oatmeal, some raisins, and some rice milk. I eat these conglomerations at least six times a week, sometimes every day. After that basic highly nutritious meal, I eat whatever comes along. My husband is a wonderful cook and likes Italian and Vietnamese food. We also eat out fairly often. I don't eat much meat, but my daily diet does include some chicken or fish or turkey. I rarely eat pastries, but indulge in hard candy.

Many books offer advice about diet and healthy eating. We must decide what works best for us. Reports show some qualms about the high protein Atkins diet and present evidence indicating it might leach calcium from the skeletal system. As we age, bone brittleness becomes a big problem.

My rule of thumb for a healthy lifestyle would be:

- Not keeping junk or fattening foods in the house. The brain sees them, or knows they are there, and a craving sets up.

- Keep lots of vegetables and fruits around to nibble for those who have an oral need to eat. Nibbling good things keep cravings at bay.

- Practice hunger now and then if you are a non-diabetic who is concerned about weight. A little hunger doesn't hurt. Then a big bunch of stir fried vegetables will seem fantastic.

- Drink lots of water. I carry water with me in the gym and keep it by my bed should I wake up.

Unfortunately, rewiring the brain to change eating addictions is more difficult than getting rid of other addictions because we must eat. We can give up smoking or drinking alcohol or using drugs and continue living. So the brain change for food takes more effort.

However, I believe that a good example of that rewiring can be seen in people who have had their stomachs stapled. They simply cannot overeat because it could kill them. At first they must struggle terribly because the food addiction is so strong. Then little rewards begin to kick in: Loss of weight; better appearance; improved ability to move around; improved self esteem. These are all brain pleasures and we want to experience more of them. Over time the way people with those stapled stomachs must eat becomes habitual and life so improves they don't want to return to their old ways.

This may not be true for every person who has had stomach-shrinking surgery because some brains are harder to work with than others. And fighting a food addiction is a struggle for anyone. But it's a worthy struggle if we can believe there's a reward: A rewired brain where food is not so important in our lives.

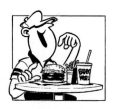

"I predict that if more people knew that a proper diet, enough sleep and exercise can increase the number of neural connections in specific regions of the brain, thereby improving memory and reasoning ability, they would take better care of themselves."
— Fred Gage, *Brain, Repair Yourself*

12 *Fitness Centers :*
The Good, The Bad, The Ugly

WANNABE EXERCISERS WILL SAY: "I could never join a gym." "Gyms are for buff, young bodies." "I would be too embarrassed."

Another reason given for avoiding gyms is the accusation that they are "meat markets." It's true that at certain times, in some fitness centers, buff, well-dressed bodies interact, intent on meeting one another, or flirting. But we don't mind watching the mating rituals of praying mantises on public television — it's biology. It's the same with the courting rituals of people. It's what humans do. Enjoy it.

An honest look around a gym would demonstrate that picture-perfect bodies are not the norm. More and more baby boomers are getting into fitness and a whole lot of gym people are not buff, picture-perfect people. Maybe they are beautiful in their own way, just not skinny model material.

Of course there will be a few conceited, haughty, self-absorbed, beautiful people but if we concentrate on our own workouts, we won't notice. Anyway, we can take comfort in the fact that their faces are going to freeze that way.

Fitness centers are valuable resources. They offer diverse equipment and classes. If one is located reasonably close to where you live or work, using it will help in building an exercise habit.

I have visited fitness centers where everyone seemed older than age 40. Some gyms are beginning to recruit older trainers because they understand that the population with money is comprised of baby boomers. In trying to recruit older members some fitness centers make the mistake of calling their offerings "programs for seniors." No one I know younger than 80 will go to a program designed for senior citizens. It conjures up wheelchair exercises in their minds.

A fitness center once recruited me to give a presentation for a special "senior citizen workshop" they were promoting to attract new members. It was a success, measured by attendance. A lot of people came. It was not a success in terms of recruitment. People came for the free stuff that was being offered, but not to join.

I prefer not giving exercise workshops to a much older population. I use examples of what happens to our bodies as we age and if everyone in the audience lives in a retirement community, what I'm talking about has already happened. It's not that those elders can't improve their health with exercise, because they can. I just can't present them with examples. As we age our muscles become stringy so the earlier we begin to build strength, the better. Older people in retirement centers already are burdened by stringy muscles.

Guidelines For Finding A Fitness Center

Here are my gym-joining guidelines for anyone who wishes to join, but feels intimidated and out of shape:

GUIDELINE NUMBER ONE: Shop around if you have some choices about location. The fitness center must be convenient for you. The chains are competing with each other and will offer new recruitment specials from time to time.

GUIDELINE NUMBER TWO: If you have decided to start with a trainer or just use the initial training offered by the gym, do not allow anyone to measure your girth with the big promise of magical results in six weeks. The more out of shape you are, the more humiliating the measuring, and six weeks just doesn't cut it. You also do not need to know your body fat ratio because you already know it's not too good and you do not need some buff, young trainer pointing that out. It totally violates the pleasure principle. Secondly, research indicates that overweight people who exercise regularly are healthier than their normal weight peers who do not exercise.

GUIDELINE NUMBER THREE: Take an honest look at the members. Everyone is not trim and beautiful. Your eyes just focus on the trim and beautiful and you don't see the real people.

GUIDELINE NUMBER FOUR: Start slowly, decide which muscles you want to strengthen, explore the weight machines fit that you. Some machines show which muscles they target. Choose the machines that target your chosen muscles. Add weight resistance gradually and carefully. Starting with too heavy weights can damage joints. Stop if you feel pain.

Start slowly with your aerobics. The pleasure will not happen if you jump on a treadmill or stationary bike, work too hard, and collapse. Collapsing does not fit my criterion of enjoying a workout.

GUIDELINE NUMBER FIVE: My most hard and fast rules concern free weights. Don't start with too heavy weights Ask someone to demonstrate the correct posture and stance. Read muscle-building magazines while standing in grocery lines to get the newest information. Do not let someone tell you to hold weights and lunge, most especially if you are a woman. Lunges put one leg ahead of the other while lowering the body. Women's knees are more susceptible to injury from lunges. I have seen trainers instruct beginners to hold weights and lunge up and down a ramp. Even young, fit women should question that. I have seen trainers instruct women to hold bar weights and squat. I have seen women squat down with weights and be unable to stand up. They are not getting stronger; they are tearing up their knees.

Don't lift weights up over your head unless you are strong, buff and want to grease up and pose. Weight lifters develop a back problem called spondylosis. The upper vertebrae come down and sort of hang over each other. Beginning to lift weights later in life could easily damage your back or knees.

I have seen trainers instruct heavy, middle-aged males, beginners, to lay on a leg press bench and push. Their stomachs are too big, their weight is cramping their innards, including their hearts, and a mighty leg push could kill them.

Concentrating on how you move, stand, sit, and feel may appear to be self-engrossed, and it is, but it's not egotistical. Compare how self-absorbed you become when you are sick or hurt.

GUIDELINE NUMBER SIX: Explore the classes. Step classes are beneficial for aerobics, movement, balance and brain exercise, but may not be inviting for beginners. Most instructors do not help the beginner become comfortable with the steps, the movements and the language that is used. I have witnessed beginners walk out in dismay, never to return because they felt awkward and embarrassed. Who can know what "walk the bench means" if they are newcomers. If a move is too strange or difficult, stand in back, march in place to keep your heart rate up. Be patient: After about five classes you will know the steps.

Power-lift classes offer to sculpt your body but are more appropriate for healthy people under age thirty. The participants lunge, squat and do overhead lifts all with weights — causing the same problems as in Guideline Five.

Most fitness centers offer a host of choices so you can explore and pick and choose what fits you: Dance classes, yoga classes, tai chi classes and many more.

GUIDELINE NUMBER SEVEN: Self-consciousness, which is so prevalent, can work against the more faint-hearted who attempt to use a gym. Even veteran gym users tend to avoid eye contact with others in the gym, unless they know them. Some people appear to be distant and cold. These people may actually be concentrating on what they are doing and do not wish to socialize, even non verbally, at that moment. The appropriate behavior is to respect those who are seriously exercising. It is rude to stare into the face of someone who's grimacing with weights. It is even more rude to stare into the face of someone who is resting between sets. That resting is an essential phase to calm the heart and muscles so the the set can be done again. For many, the resting becomes a reverie.

Accept the self-consciousness you feel. You probably won't see the people in the gym anywhere else in your life anyway. Most exercising bodies are ordinary and less-than-ordinary. If we goof up, drop a weight, are conscious of our own body flaws, it doesn't matter. Everyone is concentrating on their own bodies and many are just as self-conscious as you are.

GUIDELINE NUMBER EIGHT: Don't go to a center expecting more help than it can give. You will be offered a short time of trainer help. But trainers come in all levels of expertise and their goal is to convince you to sign up for more training hours. Staff turnover in many gyms is high. At times the overhead music is annoyingly loud. But some patrons like it. I use a portable CD with a headset so I can listen to what I like.

Recent studies demonstrate the benefits of exercising to music, but also be cautious about the effect of head sets on hearing. I suggest having a hearing exam for a baseline then using a head set that has a nub, not one that cover the whole ear canal. The nub can be placed on the upper ear and even behind the ear. After six months to a year have your hearing rechecked to be sure you have experienced no hearing loss.

Don't become obsessive about guidelines or rules, even mine or your own. It can lead to brain freeze and thwart the development of your mind games. Fitness centers are a resource; they're not perfect. You can use what fits you as you see fit.

13 *Results Of My Project*

CURIOSITY WAS THE FIRST IMPETUS for this odyssey on my personal aging path. All the studies and readings claimed that if we did thus and so for a long time we would be healthier and stronger during our later years. Then, while working in my profession, fear kicked in. Over time however, the sheer challenge of a healthy lifestyle became fun. Exhilaration followed on the heels of obvious results, especially after turning 65. At age 70 I love playing basketball. Now the challenge is exploring ways to convince others.

The information is available, but most people do not follow the advice given. Fear doesn't work either. Just consider that heart transplant patient taking up smoking the day after surgery. Pointing out the error of his ways would only make him defensive. Just as pointing out the error of my ways in any matter would make me defensive. Saying "do as I do" doesn't work either. My hope is that this book does not appear to be an ego trip but will become an inspiration for those who know that their later years can be golden if they start down the right path.

That path was demonstrated on national television when author and cardiologist Dr. Mehmet C. Oz digitally demonstrated how he would look at age 72 if he lived a healthy lifestyle. He then reversed the process and projected his appearance if he did not. The differences were striking. At this writing I'm not quite 72, but by making the right choices and running with them I believe I have demonstrated those possibilities thus far. The proof will be revealed when I am 90 years of age, but I am in no hurry to get there.

FIRST RESULT:

Not long after my 65th birthday I was in a grocery store to pick up a bottle of sparkling apple cider in a champagne bottle for a toast at a non-alcoholic party. In line, dressed in sweatshirt and sweatpants and slouched back leaning on the wall, I was fascinated with the clerk's fingernails, which were artfully done. She seemed cross. When it came to my turn, she didn't look at me, she pointed to the champagne bottle and said, "If there's alcohol in that you must show me some ID." Stunned, I said, "Uhh! It's apple cider." She picked up the bottle, looked at it, slammed it down and said, "Well you're OK then." I handed her the money and walked away still waiting for the other shoe to fall.

I couldn't compute. I kept thinking it must be similar to those times when a friendly waiter sometimes kids and says, "I'll need to see some ID, young lady." But she wasn't friendly or kidding. just crabby.

My husband was waiting at the end of the counter and kept saying, "Go back and show her your ID." I kept going because it did not make sense.

She hadn't really looked closely at me. Yet she may have seen us when we first arrived at the grocery store: I was riding on the back of the grocery cart as my husband was pushing. Whatever it was, when I got over my surprise, I told the world. This episode may not count as a result, but it helps make a point.

SECOND RESULT

I can play basketball. One granddaughter, 11 years old, will play basketball with me. A grandson had always wanted to play until he turned 13, when he didn't want his friends to notice. It is not our faces that necessarily make us seem old, it's how our bodies move through space. Older adults who walk with frailty are treated differently from those who walk firmly and upright. Walking feebly seems to prompt us to speak to adults as if they were children.

THIRD RESULT:

I am able to go to a weight machine right after a young man has used it, set the weight heavier and do the exercise without making a face. All the time in my head I'm thinking, "I'm stronger than you are." That may not be a legitimate result but it gives me pleasure and spurs me on.

FOURTH RESULT:

At times, after a day of heavy exercise and a lot of work, I go to bed early and and am able to sleep for 10 hours without waking up. I need the sleep to catch up. Bless those kegels.

FIFTH RESULT:

Once a year I have a complete physical. I like going because doctors always act surprised when entering the room. I fractured my ankle this year running in the dark, on the sidewalk, in sandal shoes. I was asked: "Is that your real age?"

I have long claimed that we all hope to live until 100, hauling water and chopping wood, and dying quietly in our sleep.

I must clarify that I am not beautiful. I do not enjoy a sexy shape. I'm more square. I recently encountered someone I hadn't seen in years and the first thing they said was, "Gosh, you took healthy." I am healthy and it shows.

SIXTH RESULT:

I can play the piano. The playing quickly hopped into my head after not touching a piano for 55 years. I will lay odds that the speed can be attributed to brain games.

SEVENTH RESULT:

I intend to take trains around Europe next year. I had never nagged my husband to begin exercising. When I renewed my fitness center membership five years ago I added him and several of our adult children. He agreed at that time, "OK, I'll go with you on Tuesdays and Thursdays." Soon he was going every day. When we were riding trains in Europe, two years after he had been going regularly to the gym, he commented several times that he would never have been able to travel that way had he not been working out. He was able to climb mountains in Italy.

My husband's result cannot be considered a part of my research project, but I will use everything I can to make a point to add to the credibility of my study.

 None of us hears a piece of music exactly the same as another. It's not that some people march to different drummers; rather, we each march to our own drum. So we may as well sit back and enjoy our differences.

RESULT NUMBER EIGHT:
  My physical results:
    Total Cholesterol: 169
    Fasting Triglicerides: 90
    Cholesterol, HDL: 53
    Cholesterol, LDL: 98
    Glucose, fasting: 86
    Bone Density: Upper Body 105%
    Bone Density: Lower Body 107%
    Blood Pressure Range (during one day):
      133/72 after a gym workout
      120/70 after lunch
      119/69 late afternoon

During one period in my life my blood pressure rose, requiring me to limit my coffee intake and meditate in an attempt to bring the reading down. It worked: There are times when my blood pressure reading is as low as 116/65.

For this continuing research the results will be measured yearly. There's no guarantee that a healthy lifestyle yields similar results for everyone. But there will be positive results for every body that is cared for with regular physical exercise, healthy eating, an active lifestyle and an active brain, just as a sedentary, unhealthy lifestyle will yield negative results.

Premature decline and frailty is preventable. Success takes some thinking ahead. It takes concentration. It takes focusing on reality. More importantly, it takes determination. You can choose. What I am advocating works for me. (So far).

> *"Wait awhile, eternity*
> *Old Mother Nature's got nothing on me."*
> — John Prine

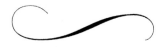

I saw the cardiologist Dr. Mehmet C. Oz on television where he digitally demonstrated how he would look at age 72 if he lived a healthy lifestyle, then how he would look if he did not. The differences were striking. I knew I had done what he was demonstrating. I have no idea how I would be now, at age 70, if I had not consciously followed a lifestyle that I had read and taught about a long time ago. I suspect I would be like Dr. Oz's second digital demonstration. Lifestyle is the big one, folks.

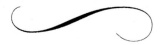

14 Conclusion:
Because Gravity Works

STIMULATING BOTH BODY AND BRAIN works to our advantage as we age. It seems a paradox that we are able to regenerate and sustain healthy cells all the while we are programmed to eventually leave this earth.

To quote Sherwin Nuland from his book *How We Die*: "Nature's job is to send us packing, medicine be damned." But with the advent of knowledge from the medical community, many of us are living a long time. Unfortunately our bodies' decline can make that added time miserable, even painful.

So, along with our natural bent toward making room for further generations, there seems to be an element in our makeup that allows for stimulated cells, both in our brains and bodies, to not only slow the decline, but to stay viable for a longer time. Our program to die seems at odds with our bodies' ability to regenerate cells and keep us going longer.

Perhaps, in between our inclination to slide into oblivion and our ability to stay healthy and keep living, we can find the middle ground of choice.

*"We want to live forever
but we know we never will."*
— Cat Stevens

99

Something in our makeup allows for a certain degree of regeneration, better health, and a longer life.

A major reward for my mother in her long-time employment was a parking space right across the street from her job. She believed that walking one, two or three blocks to her car, after sitting at a desk all day, was doing her in. She lived in a time when mothers stayed in the hospital for two weeks after having a baby and exercise was felt to be too much exertion. Later in life she worried herself sick over my exercising.

Evolution of thought takes some strange twists and turns and, because of research on the aging process, we now know my mother's theories of resting and never exercising were not only incorrect, those beliefs were not healthy.

For as long as possible, our bodies require movement and our minds require involvement. But some strange pleasure quirk in the evolution of our brains makes us cling to the easier road. And what feeds that sedentary pleasure quirk in the short run denies us a lot of living for the long run.

Like the example of my mother's job, it's easier to rest after sitting all day than it is to walk to get our blood circulating. Sedentary jobs are subtly tiring. Otherwise, why are we exhausted after sitting in an office for 8 hours, then feel as if we need to rest? Maybe our energy systems have been thwarted because our blood hasn't been moving.

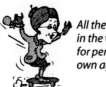

All the medical breakthroughs in the world can never substitute for personal responsibility for our own aging.

100

It's that inertia difficulty that keeps us from moving our bodies, getting our blood circulating, keeping our bones strong, avoiding depression, and even fighting some forms of cancer. That difficulty is a barrier and we can discover ways to get up and over a barrier. If scare tactics work, then scare tactics are necessary. If pointing out the fallacy of excuses works, then jumping on excuses is necessary.

If the search for joy and a different type of pleasure motivates you, then go for it. We will be better served if mental and physical exercise can evolve as a way of life. Starting that way of life can be difficult: It's always easier to rest than to push our bodies to move.

Our brains maximize a learned skill into a less alert part of consciousness so it eventually fires at a lower level of activity. We begin to do so many things at that level of consciousness that most of what we do becomes a habit and our brains slide into cruise state and early decline. But stimulate those brains with new experiences and learning and they stay alive and kicking.

The same goes for our bodies. Neglect a muscle and it withers. Look at what becomes of muscle that is locked into a cast when a bone is broken. It shrinks. It must be built up to recover to it's former state. It can recover.

It takes effort to stand up and stride with vigor. It's a small thing, but over time, our bodies form in the way we move them. Forcing our bodies to look and act healthy has strong effects on how we feel at any age, but especially in our later years. Once we restore health to our bodies, staying erect not only seems effortless, it becomes habit.

All the medical breakthroughs in the world can never substitute for personal responsibility for our own aging. If we haven't exercised our hearts and lungs and legs and a crisis forces us to run quickly, medical know-how won't help us. If we are in poor shape our bodies could fail from the sudden exertion.

Imagine chicken little is screaming, "the sky is falling," and you realize you must run for half an hour to save your life. Could you do it? If we're physically fit our bodies will shrug their shoulders and find a long run or a sustained sprint in a crisis to be no big deal.

Aging is a more profound exertion than any sudden crisis. Being unnecessarily locked into a dependent, frail body when we could have done something to prevent it is the crisis. Being obese may not be an issue at age 40 but, at age 75, trying to locate caregivers who can help get us on our feet — and it would take more than one person — is a crisis issue.

So often we hear of the need to legislate more care for the elderly, or the need to find cures for age-related ailments, or the importance of allowing frail elders to make as many choices on their own as possible. Allowing choice is not the same as having the ability to make choices on our own. The opportunity to make independent choices in our later years depends on how we live now. With each of us looking toward our personal futures, we have some voice in the ability to walk out of the care home after a visit, or watching our more healthy, vigorous friends do the walking after visiting us in our care home.

We have used our powerful minds to thwart nature because we fear death. And we have thwarted nature in various ways, including living longer and staying stronger into older age. That is, some of us stay healthier and stronger — but a whole lot of us just live longer.

We often hear the lament that society only focuses on the young and that our population treats the elderly differently than younger adults. But biology drives that discrimination, not selfishness. Nature set us up so we are attracted to younger, stronger bodies for procreation; then we are supposed to wither and die to make room for the new people. A strong, vital older person is treated differently than a frail, dependent elder, because the frail person's body language sends a message that they need attentive care. We want to counter that perception of helplessness for our own later years.

We can't be so foolish as to believe that every person in a care home could have prevented their situation with a certain lifestyle. Unforeseen things happen and we can encounter undesirable consequences in living, including outcomes determined by our personal genetics. But we now know that a large percentage of the physical dependency related to age could have been prevented had dependent people known the facts, and if they had lived a vital lifestyle — a lifestyle that counters age-related problems.

There's so much evidence that demonstrates we are able to become healthier, stronger, and in more control of our destiny as we age. Healthy, strong bodies let our hearts and lungs pump easily without stress. If our heart and lungs are working well, our circulation is better. If our circulation is better we not only look good, our brain is getting the oxygen it needs. If our bodies are working well our self-esteem is higher. But it's getting from sedentary to the discovery of the beauty and strength of our bodies that is the key.

It requires reasonable goals, and the determination to develop our own individuality enough so we know what we can do, what we can expect of our body, and are able to ignore negative comparisons.

I possess a short, square body and I do revel in my strength. But sometimes I see a young, shapely, beautiful young woman in the gym, and think, "I wish I could look like that." But I didn't look like that when I was twenty years old. After that brief reverie, I go back to appreciating what I can do. It was just a quick negative comparison.

We may live a long time and barring unforeseen accidents, the time required in our lives now to maintain a healthy body is nothing compared to the time that can be spent later in dependency.

Building a healthy lifestyle is circular: We feel our uniqueness, we begin exercising and eating better. That lifestyle change raises our sense of well being. As our self-esteem raises, our ability to exercise and maintain a healthier diet becomes easier and more enjoyable, and we relish our uniqueness. The more enjoyable we find our lives, the more little surprises we experience along the say. The more little surprises, the higher our self esteem. There is no magic pill. There is, however, the possibility of a gold medal for the willing.

Barring the fickle finger of fate, and thanks to medical technology, you have won the chance at a longer life than your ancestors. For many, that added time can allow for an opportunity to experience some diverse lifestyles. What you choose to do will have a tremendous impact on those lifestyle opportunities.

104

So if you have experienced the epiphany and are determined to find pleasure and habit with an improved lifestyle, remember:

- Start where you are without criticizing your body — it prefers to be loved.

- Begin with what you can do now. You are competing with life, not other people.

- Keep it simple. Make it fun.

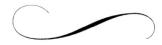

"So be sure when you step,
Step with care and great tact
and remember that life's a great balancing act.
Just never forget to be dexterous and deft,
And never mix up your right foot with your left."

— Dr. Seuss

105

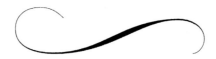

We can't be so foolish as to believe that every person in a care home could have prevented their situation with a certain lifestyle. Unforeseen things happen and we can encounter undesirable consequences in living, including outcomes determined by our personal genetics. But we now know that a large percentage of the physical dependency related to age could have been prevented had dependent people known the facts, and if they had lived a vital lifestyle — a lifestyle that counters age-related problems.

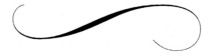

Bibliography

Andes, Karen, *A Woman's Book Of Strength* (Perigee Books, 1995).

Dr. Seuss, *Oh, The Places You'll Go!* (Random House, 1990).

Gage, Fred, "Brain, Repair Yourself" in *Scientific American: Better Brains** (Sept. 2003).

Gerish, Michael, *When Working Out Isn't Working Out* (St. Martin S. Griffin, 1999).

Goldberg, Linn, M.D. & Diane L. Elliot, M.D., *The Healing Power Of Exercise* (Wiley, 2000).

Helmstetter, Shad, *The Self Talk Solution* (Pocket Books, 1987).

Horgan, John, *The Undiscovered Mind* (The Free Press, 1999).

Hyman, Steven, "Diagnosing Disorders" in *Scientific American: Better Brains** (Sept. 2003).

Johnson, Steven, *Mind Wide Open* (Scribner, 2004).

K•I•S•S, *Guide To Yoga* (DK Publishing, Inc., 2001).

Knoops, Kim T. B., MsC, et al, "Mediterranian Diet, Lifestyle Factors, and 10-Year Mortality in Elderly European Men and Women: The HALE Project", *Journal of the American Medical Association*, vol. 292, no. 12, September 22, 2004, pp. 1433-1439.

Kotulak, Ronald & Peter Gorner, *Aging On Hold* (Tribune Publishing, 1992).

Nelson, Mirian, Ph.D. & Wernick, Sarah, Ph.D., *Strong Women Stay Strong* (Bantam Books, 1997).

Nuland, Sherwin, *How We Die* (Vintage Books, 1993).

Nuland, Sherwin, *The Wisdom Of The Body* (Alfred A. Knopf, 1997).

Oz, Mehmet C., *Healing from the Heart: A Leading Surgeon Combines Eastern and Western Traditions to Create the Medicine of the Future* (Plume, 1999).

Quartz, Steven, Ph. D. & Terrence Sejnowski, Ph. D., *Liars, Lovers, and Heroes* (Morrow, 2002).

Restak, Richard, M.D., *Mozart's Brain and the Fighter Pilot: Unleashing Your Brain's Potential* (Three Rivers Press, 2001). (Considered a personal trainer for the brain).

Restak, Richard, M.D., *The New Brain* (Rodale Press, 2003).

Restak, Richard, M.D., *The Brain Has A Mind Of It's Own* (Crown Publishers, 1991).

Rickells, Robert, & Caleb Finch, *Aging: A Natural History* (Scientific American Library, 1995).

Roizen, Michael, *Real Age* (Cliff Street Books, 1999).

Rowe, John, M.D. & Robert Kahn, Ph.D., *Successful Aging* (Dell Publishing, 1998).

Scaravelli, Vanda, *Awakening The Spine* (Harper Collins, 1991).

Snowdon, David, Ph.D., *Aging With Grace* (Bantam Books, 2001).

Warshofsky, Fred, *Stealing Time: The New Science of Aging* (TV Books, 1999)

Weeks, David, M.D. & Jamie James, *Secrets Of The Super Young* (Villard Books, 1998).

*NOTE Scientific American Special Issues:
"Better Brains" (September 2003, $10.95) can be ordered at *Scientific American*, Dept. BBS03. 415 Madison Ave. NY 10017, or online at <<www.orderissues@sciam.com>>.

"Mind — The Brain — A Look Inside" (January 2004) *Scientific American*, Dept. Mind. P.O Box 10067 Des Moines, IA 50340
Order any back issue of *Scientific American* online at:
<<http://m1.buysub.com/webapp/wcs/stores/servlet/CategoryDisplay?catalo gId=11001&storeId=11001&categoryId=10092&langId=-1>>.

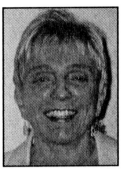

Thelma J. Lofquist

T. J. Lofquist started her college education, at the age of 37, as a single parent of six children. In graduate school her two fields of study became Environmental Psychology and Gerontology. While at the university she took dance classes, then wrote her Master's thesis using jazz dance as therapy. Her experiences both dancing and teaching classes on physical activity and aging prompted her to explore the effects of lifestyle on the aging process. While writing her doctoral thesis she began assessing elder care facilities and made referrals to families of frail elders. Counseling those families led to her book, *Frail Elders and the Wounded Caregiver* (Binford & Mort).

Healthy lifestyle, coupled with Dr. Lofquist's fascination with the many wonders of recent brain research, has prompted her to write a new book, *I Don't Want To Be Old When I Get Old.*

She writes a regular monthly column, "Exercise Is A State Of Mind," conducts exercise workshops, teaches jazz dance, and presents talks on "The Healthy Brain and How To Enhance It."

The research shows clearly that many chronic aches and pains, and dependency of older age, can be thwarted with lifestyle changes. When we discover and apply this information we not only will reward our own later lives, we will help our children as well by extending our ability to live independently.

Dr. Lofquist has learned and is learning the value of walking the talk, and strongly believes that it is incumbent upon all of us to take charge of our own aging.

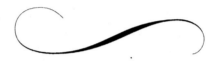

"You do the fitness often enough and something marvelous happens. You and the fitness become one. Finally, the fitness does you."
— Richard Restak, M. D., neurologist and author
of *Mozart's Brain and the Fighter Pilot*

Printed in the United States
35513LVS00007B/134